birth stories

birth
stories

Katrina O'Brien

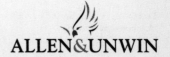

For Joe and Rosalie

First published in 2005

Copyright © Katrina O'Brien 2005

All rights reserved. No part of this book may be reproduced or transmitted in any form or by any means, electronic or mechanical, including photocopying, recording or by any information storage and retrieval system, without prior permission in writing from the publisher. The *Australian Copyright Act 1968* (the Act) allows a maximum of one chapter or 10 per cent of this book, whichever is the greater, to be photocopied by any educational institution for its educational purposes provided that the educational institution (or body that administers it) has given a remuneration notice to Copyright Agency Limited (CAL) under the Act.

Allen & Unwin
83 Alexander Street
Crows Nest NSW 2065
Australia
Phone: (61 2) 8425 0100
Fax: (61 2) 9906 2218
Email: info@allenandunwin.com
Web: www.allenandunwin.com

National Library of Australia
Cataloguing-in-Publication entry:

Birth stories.

ISBN 1 74114 339 X.

1. Childbirth - Anecdotes. 2. Childbirth - Popular works.
3. Childbirth - Psychological aspects. 4. Mother and child.
I. O'Brien, Katrina.

618.40922

Typeset in 13/15pt Bembo by Midland Typesetters,
Maryborough, Victoria
Printed in Australia by McPherson's Printing Group

10 9 8 7 6 5 4 3 2 1

Contents

Introduction	1
Jane Torley 'Tell Mum to wait until half-time'	10
Linda Burney Completing the jigsaw	26
Anne Stanley The short distance between life and death	39
Nikki Gemmell 'I felt like a she-wolf who'd gone to the hills'	55
Sally Machin My great unknown adventure	70
Jenny Ann Cook Into his arms	87
Penny McCarthy The perfect family	102
Kirsty Sword Gusmão Mascot for a nation	121
Snezna Kerekovic 'I had a choice and I chose a Caesarean'	139
Amanda Keller A very public pregnancy	152
Alison Baker 'Mummy's tummy's broken'	168
Zali Steggall 'So much for a birth plan!'	186
Liz Scott 'The greatest high I had ever experienced'	202
Katrina O'Brien 'I thought I was risking my baby's life'	216
Acknowledgments	230
About the author	232

Introduction

Ask a woman about the day (or night) she gave birth and you are bound to hear a gripping story filled with drama, suspense, elation, joy and possibly sadness. Don't ask and you'll probably never hear it.

Birth is one of the most profound experiences a woman is likely to go through, but unless you are sitting in a mothers' group surrounded by screaming newborns, you are unlikely to hear the details. Whether it's a symptom of women too busy getting on with their lives or a reluctance to share stories that are deemed too personal, the stark realities of giving birth largely remain a mystery.

Well, not any more.

As a journalist, I have always been intrigued by deeply human stories, and what could be more human than giving birth? Put a woman who is normally in control of every aspect of her life into a situation she has never been in before and a story soon unfolds. Throw in her desires, her fears, her best-laid plans, the shock of pain like no other, the unexpected, the absurd and the desperately emotional, and you've got a compelling read.

I've always loved hearing the details of other women's birth experiences but it took a conversation in the middle of 2003 with my then three-year-old son Joe to realise how intriguing these stories could be. As I sat on the edge of the bath and re-told the story of his birth—it was a favourite at the time—I suddenly realised how different it was to the story I would one day tell his little sister, Rosalie, when she eventually found the words to ask.

I'd always considered myself a bit of an obstetrics case study—the births of my two children being so completely different—but it was only when I had the luxury of recalling the details that the differences became so obvious.

Later that night, in the haze just before sleep, I decided that my story—along with many other women's—was worth telling. I instantly came up with a list of 23 women who I knew had intriguing stories to share, and scribbled down their names on the back of an envelope—one I still carry around in my diary—along with the premise of my idea.

The concept went like this: take a group of women back to one of the most intimate events of their lives, a time when they were at their most vulnerable—and powerful—and get to the core of what happened. Ask them what went right, what went wrong, and why they chose the paths they did. Basically, go into their minds and bodies as they birthed and find out how they reacted to the enormity of facing their most primal selves and an irrepressible life-force—whether squatting in a birthing pool or lying in an operating theatre.

I wanted the real stories—the highs and the lows—and not just the bits that might later turn into 'horror stories' or 'war stories' or 'badges of honour'. And I wanted these women to tell their stories in their own words to capture the intensity of the experience.

I'd read my share of birth and pregnancy books, but had never come across a book that purely told the stories of women giving birth. I'd always found the tiny snippets of women's stories in these guidebooks much more intriguing than the oblique medical descriptions and two-dimensional illustrations. Maybe it's the intrinsic stickybeak in me, but I wanted to know more and wondered why these powerfully moving—and very significant—women's stories weren't being recorded. I knew birth, like life, was not restricted to textbook anecdotes. I also had a sneaking suspicion other women would be interested too.

When I spoke about my idea to others, I found I was right. TV and radio host Amanda Keller remembers: 'I used to go and see my obstetrician in the eastern suburbs of Sydney. All these women would be sitting there, a lot of them in suits, and I'd think, "This obstetrician must see all of us with our day faces on, and then see us at our most animal." It must be extraordinary.'

I also wondered why there was still so much secrecy and silence surrounding birth. My mother, who gave birth to three daughters in the late 1960s, avoided discussing anything about her births—even as I waited, at the age of 31, for the arrival of my first child. The fragments I'd hear were from my father: he'd recall how he'd left my labouring mother lying on a bed holding her rosary beads. Visiting hours were over—there was no such thing as having a husband present at a birth—and I think she thought she was going to die.

My auntie Claire, who had three children in the 1950s and 1960s, thought she'd wet herself when her waters broke and had absolutely no idea what she was in for when she arrived at hospital to have her first baby. A nun told her to get undressed and then left the room. When she came back in, Claire was sitting there naked and was told: 'You may be pregnant, but do you think you could show some degree of modesty?' Luckily for her, the birth 'was an absolute breeze', she says.

We're not in the last century and we have the Internet and a plethora of birth guides now, but somehow birth is still in the domain of 'you'll find out when you get there'. Many first-time mothers crave knowledge about birth—women who wouldn't dream of going into a work meeting or job interview unprepared—but because they are working or might be the first pregnant woman amongst friends, rarely come across new mothers. Even if they want to hear about the reality of birth through the stories of others, they can't. Instead, they sit around antenatal classes as clueless as the next woman.

Of course, none of us can adequately describe to another how a contraction will feel, how your body will burn when the baby arrives at the entrance to your birth canal, or explain the sensation of putting a newborn's wanton mouth to your breast for the first time. But by sharing stories of just some of the things that can happen during birth, it is possible to gain a degree of insight into the unknown.

I began my search for stories soon after that conversation with Joe. As the months went by, my list of prospective subjects extended to more than 130 and I soon realised the difficulty would come in cutting this number down. Each of these women—and I knew there were many more—had a very good reason to be in this collection. Every birth story is fascinating and intrinsically unique, as every woman who has had a child births in a deeply personal way and reacts to the joys and adversities in a manner that is all her own.

There is no way *Birth Stories* could ever be completely conclusive, nor could it cover all the eventualities and outcomes of birth—it covers only some. When narrowing down my collection, I decided to include as diverse a range as I could, each having a very specific reason to be here. I wanted to highlight the choices women have today. I was also determined to show that there were many ways to have a baby.

I didn't set out to prove that one way of giving birth was better than another. One high-profile mother I contacted expressed interest in being interviewed, but only if the book would be pro-natural. But that wasn't what *Birth Stories* was about. This book was about showing that women do have options and that sometimes even the best-laid plans and intentions can unravel at the most inappropriate times.

Birth isn't a medical procedure, but for many women it can be, often by choice. Australia has an incredibly high intervention rate, with more than one in four women giving birth by Caesarean (27 per cent in 2002, according to the National Perinatal Statistics Unit), and although many would agree that this is a less than ideal situation, the women who do have highly intervened births cannot be ignored. Nor should they be made to feel that their birth experiences were in any way less significant or sound than others.

Many women also suffer from terrible grief when they are unable to have the birth experience they desperately desired. One woman told me how she cried as she checked into hospital for the elective Caesarean she didn't want to have for her second child. She'd had an emergency Caesarean with her first baby after more than a day of induced labour and after her pelvis was deemed too small to deliver vaginally. Her obstetrician couldn't understand it, but she longed to deliver naturally the second time. He recommended a Caesarean at 38 weeks. She negotiated 40 weeks in the hope she would spontaneously go into labour, and spent the day before her Caesarean power-walking and emotionally distressed. 'On all the case notes and baby health centre referrals it was written down as an elective Caesarean, and technically it was,' she says. 'But it wasn't to me. It was a scheduled Caesarean. I would have much preferred a natural birth.'

Another spoke of her feelings of inadequacy when a man she knew boasted about his partner being 'designed to have babies' after giving birth to their two children without drugs and with very short labours. This woman had just recovered from a traumatic birth experience: not in the birth centre she longed to give birth in, but in the delivery suite. A vacuum pull had been necessary and her baby ended up in intensive care.

Rather than make women feel that they will have somehow failed if they don't get the birth experience they desire, I wanted to tell a variety of stories to show that all birth experiences are equally valid—and that these women are not alone.

I also wanted to show that women have choices. With the potent mix of increased medical insurance coverage, high intervention rates, and an indemnity crisis in Australia that has forced many independent midwives and obstetricians out of business, it can feel that birth choices in this country are becoming increasingly limited. And for a first-time labouring woman who enters a delivery suite and has her bulging tummy strapped to heart-rate and contraction monitors, the notion of choice can seem completely non-existent.

But women do have choices. There are slowly increasing numbers of midwife-centric services attached to hospitals where women with low-risk pregnancies can have continuous care from the same midwife. And there are very early moves within New South Wales to make publicly funded home births possible, a system which already exists in New Zealand, where home births account for between 7 and 10 per cent of births, according to the New Zealand College of Midwives.

Even within the standard hospital system there are still choices to be made along each turn on the journey towards birth: from the doctors and/or hospitals we choose (and the questions we ask), the centres we decide to give birth in, whether or not to labour longer than our medical practitioners might prefer, when to be given our babies post-birth, or even how soon to have that epidural. It took more than one birth for some of the women in *Birth Stories* to realise they had choices, while others exercised their rights from the moment they conceived.

Birth in itself is amazing—yet put in the context of a woman's life, it becomes compelling. For many of the women of *Birth Stories*, having a baby was about so much more than control and whether or not to use drugs for pain relief. One mother explained to me how she was told at the age of 14 that she would never have children, while another recounted feeling grief rather than joy after the birth of her baby boy. These, I felt, were stories which needed to be told.

As I sat up in the loneliest hour of night feeding my newly born Rosalie in early 2002, I remember finding it incredibly grounding to be aware that on the other side of the world, actress Cate Blanchett was possibly doing the same with her new son. Birth is the great equaliser, and even the most high-profile mother with access to the best in nannies, political power and modern medicine must go through the same experience every other mother does. She faces the pain, the dilemmas and the leaking breasts afterwards, and that's why you'll recognise some of the names in *Birth Stories*.

I spent many hours speaking to women about their birth experiences. I sat in their kitchens and lounge rooms, spoke to them on the phone at midnight while children slept, talked at the beginning of mid-afternoon naps as newborn twins hummed their way to sleep, and in the offices of Sydney's Parliament House. I felt incredibly privileged to be invited into these extraordinary women's lives and homes as they relived some of their most private moments, and was amazed and thrilled at how candidly and eloquently they spoke.

For many, it was the first time they'd sat down and verbalised their feelings about an experience that will stay with them forever. Retelling their stories took them back to a time when life revolved around them and their needs and wants—before it all shifted to that grizzly little creature sleeping at the end of the bed, a little creature who suddenly turned into a toddler and then a teenager.

Sometimes the rawness and intensity of these memories took my breath away. At other times we laughed and laughed. It's amazing how the most banal and basic experience can bring out the ridiculous. A vegetable strainer to catch poos, anyone?

The more I spoke with women about birth, the more

I realised that the concept of a birth plan needs to be updated. Sure, we can read and research as much as possible and have an idea about what we might like to happen. But for many, there is no way of knowing how they will react when faced with the pain of labour and the rollercoaster that birth can be.

Of course, there are exceptions. Many women are determined to birth without pain relief or even in silence and manage to do both successfully. But others with the best intentions may be forced to make vast turnarounds to their plans and be left floored by the experience. I've come to realise that in birth it's probably best to be prepared for the unexpected.

I have also discovered exactly how much women like to be in control. And while one woman's idea of control is handing her body over to a surgeon to cut through her uterus, another's is having medical staff completely removed from the process. But facing the shock of a newborn is when most of the women of *Birth Stories* found their lives totally out of control. Luckily, they have lived to tell the tale.

Birth Stories is filled with very personal stories and is not intended as a medical guide to giving birth. Nor is it intended to act as contraception, as my sister-in-law has suggested. It is a recollection of events seen through the eyes of the women who were centrally involved. I hope that their stories will entertain, empower and enlighten—and demystify the emotionally and physically challenging event that is birth.

'Tell Mum to wait until half-time'

JANE TORLEY

I was just 16 when I fell pregnant in 1986. My mother had recently pulled me out of school and packed me off to relatives because she thought I was setting a bad example for my younger siblings. When I told my parents I was pregnant, they said, 'Right, you can leave now.'

We were Catholic and there was so much shame. There was also a lot of pressure on me to have an abortion. It was very traumatic, but when you're young, you respond to everything very quickly. I never planned on being a young mother—I was working in a Canberra florist and had ideas about what I wanted to do—but everything changed once I found out I was pregnant. *Well, I'm going to be a mum*, I thought. *I've got to sort myself out.* The child was my life now, so whatever plans I had were on the backburner.

Paul and I had been going out for 18 months and I was madly in love with him. I knew we'd be together forever, although he wasn't so sure. He was only 21, which was very young to have this sort of responsibility, but he was very supportive and we soon moved in together.

I didn't have much support from anywhere else though. It was quite strange. I still felt like a teenager but I wasn't able to do all those teenage things and other teenagers thought, *Oh dear, she's gone the next step and got herself into trouble.* And all the adults frowned on me because I was in trouble, so I was sort of in-between.

None of my relatives would talk to me about my pregnancy—it really was a taboo subject. It was as if, 'Yes, you've got to have had sex to have fallen pregnant, but hey, we're not going to talk about the birth because it all just seems a little bit too rude.' But I wanted to talk about it. *Look, I've done the rude stuff,* I thought. *Now can we just get down to it?*

I wasn't ashamed and Paul and I were happy in our little oasis. The people I worked with were really nice and just accepted me, but whenever we came out of isolation and into contact with our parents, reality hit and it became difficult. We coped though, and just accepted that that was the way it had to be.

I went to see my local GP throughout the pregnancy. I don't know if teenagers get the same treatment today, but nothing at all was explained to me. I'd go in and he'd weigh me. 'You're right,' he'd say. 'Goodbye.' He didn't tell me anything about what was going to happen or what I needed to do and I didn't really know where to go to find out. My aunt sent me a very old-fashioned birth book towards the end of the pregnancy. When the baby's due, have your bag packed and off you go to hospital, it said. But I wanted to know what happened when I got there.

My GP did mention that there were classes available but he advised me to take my partner. Paul worked shifts as a telephonist and I knew he wouldn't be able to come, so I didn't go. And I naively thought that giving birth at my age would be easy and natural.

I took a week off work before the baby was due and the contractions came right on time on the morning of 27 July 1987. Paul and I went straight to the hospital, which was five minutes' drive away. 'No, you're not in labour,' said the midwife. 'Go home.' So we went home but the pain became unbelievable. I started flapping around the house like a bird and a couple of hours later we were back in the hospital.

I was there for hours and hours and the doctor eventually came in and broke my waters. They worked out the baby was the wrong way around, in a posterior position, and it was just so painful so they gave me the gas. But I began hallucinating. My grandfather was a World War II prisoner of war and I started going on about troops and war and talking to the medical staff about Nazis.

It was all quite terrifying and the next thing I knew they were giving me an epidural. They didn't ask me if I wanted one, they just did it, and that was the worst thing in the world because I had no control over my body at all.

I was so young and it really felt like the doctors and nurses were just doing what they wanted. I didn't know I had choices. I just did everything I was told to do. I didn't want to rock the boat so I didn't say a word.

Paul kept on going out for a cigarette and I just about killed him each time he came back in because I really felt alone. And then when it came to pushing out the baby—

more than 25 hours after going into labour—all these student doctors and nurses came in to watch. I knew it was a teaching hospital but there was no consultation whatsoever. It felt like a million people were there and I found it all so humiliating.

The doctor used forceps to get the baby out and I didn't feel anything except for the click of my hips, which was constant. It was an awful sensation and I didn't know what was going on, but I could see the doctor: he had his foot up on the bed, and was just pulling and pulling. My parents had a farm and sometimes calves died inside the cows and my father would have to pull them out with a tractor and I kept on envisioning that. I really thought the baby's head was going to come off its shoulders.

It was so awful and I was terrified. *I've got to get over this hurdle*, I kept thinking. *There's a baby at the end of all this effort.*

The doctor eventually pulled the baby out. The forceps had taken off a layer of skin from around the baby's neck, so he really was quite a mess. The midwife gave him to me briefly—I was so relieved he was breathing and fine—and then she took him away. 'He needs a bath now,' she said. And Robert was gone.

Paul soon left to celebrate and smoke a cigar. Mum turned up briefly and also left. Robert was jaundiced so they took him to neonatal intensive care and I was taken away and put in a dementia ward because the maternity one was full. It was awful. I felt abandoned and all I kept thinking was, *When do I get my baby back?* I still had the epidural in so I couldn't walk around to the nursery and it was 24 hours before I saw my baby again.

After any birth there's a let-down eventually, but at least these days you're left with the baby and it's wonderful. But Robert was born in the days before newborns stayed in the room with their mothers, so I was left there without my baby, feeling traumatised by the whole experience, and it was such a huge let-down.

I was sleep deprived for much of the seven days I was in hospital, but when Robert and I left, I never looked back. I moved on pretty quickly but in a lot of ways it put me off ever having another child. I probably should have had some counselling after Robert's birth—it was so traumatic—but nobody was interested in talking about it. Most of the doctors just wanted to talk about the facts on paper.

Eventually I went and did some research and realised there were different ways to give birth. But the whole experience made me incredibly wary of the medical profession and when I became pregnant with my second child two years later—this time it was planned—I knew I would do things my way and have a natural birth.

I was very overweight when I had Robert and thought that might have had something to do with me not handling the birth, so I put myself on a strict diet this time around and approached the birth very self-consciously.

I decided to go to an obstetrician, and on my first visit I made it clear I didn't want any drugs during the birth. This time I was very vocal. 'I don't want an epidural, I don't want gas, I don't want pethidine, I don't want anything,' I raved. 'Okay,' he said. 'You've obviously had a bad experience.' On the second visit, he told me he'd be doing an internal examination the next time I came in, and as I walked home I starting thinking and came to a conclusion. *Nope*, I thought. *I'm not going to him any more.*

My reaction was totally out of the blue but I knew I didn't want anyone touching me again unless my baby was coming out. I booked myself into the hospital and went cold turkey and refused to see him again. I decided I would follow my own health routine: I would weigh myself, keep a little book of what I was doing physically and if I ever got sick, I'd just go to my GP. I wasn't going to have any more of people telling me what to do.

Paul thought I'd lost my marbles. 'You can't do this,' he said. 'You need to go and see someone.' But I was very definite. I'd made a choice and wasn't going to talk about it any more.

The baby was four days late so I went to my GP. He was shocked when he saw me. 'The baby's late,' I said. 'Aren't you seeing an obstetrician?' he asked. 'No,' I replied. 'I think we'd better organise for you to see one and I want you back here in a week,' he said. He was very understanding. He'd seen that I'd had another baby and guessed that I'd had a bad experience, but I wasn't about to tell him how badly that first birth had affected me. Too many emotions would have come up and I didn't want to let that monster out.

I agreed to go to the obstetrician but it wasn't necessary because four days later I went into labour. Robert's labour had all been in the back, but this pain was in the front and was much more subtle. I didn't want to rush into the hospital, so I went and had a bath. The labour felt like more of a gentle bearing down, but I still flapped my arms at 60 miles an hour and breathed really quickly.

Paul became anxious after a little while. 'Come on,' he said. 'You'd better get in there.' He was very keen to go to that hospital—he likes to get the births over with and is not one of those men who want to cut the umbilical cord or anything like that.

We eventually got to the hospital and the doctor, who was a very gentle man, stayed back and watched while the midwife delivered Kayler. The labour was only three hours all up and it was a totally different experience from that first one. I didn't have any drugs—there was no way I was going to lose control of myself or my body ever again—and the midwives were wonderful and incredibly supportive.

It was only two and half years since I'd had Robert in that same hospital, but the whole system had changed by then. Kayler slept in my room and there was none of that awful separation that I had with Robert.

I turned 20 a month after Kayler was born and we definitely decided that two was good for us. I went back to work at the florist and Paul did his Higher School Certificate. Afterwards he started up a gardening business that kept him really busy and we were married in March 1995.

Then, when I was 25, I became pregnant with our third child. It really was a surprise, but we were both happy about it. *Well*, I thought, *it doesn't matter how many children we have now.*

This time I had shared care between my GP and the hospital and I was very happy with that. I went into labour a week early and because the baby was posterior and pushing on my back just as during Robert's labour, the pain was incredibly intense. 'I've got to get out of this pain,' I said, not long after arriving at the hospital, and they kept asking me if I wanted relief. But drugs just weren't an option for me. 'Nope,' I'd say. 'No relief.'

My midwife gave me hot packs to put on my back and suggested I rotate from one side to the other and within about half an hour, the baby turned around. It was so nice to get that baby into the birth canal. *Thank God*, I thought.

The birth was very good and when we brought Michael home I thought maybe we'd have another one. I'm very maternal and have always been a big fan of babies, so I was pregnant with our fourth child within a year.

Nicola's birth was very similar to Michael's. She was a week and a half early and like the others was in a posterior position. The labour was three hours long and we made it to the hospital with only an hour to spare. Luckily, the hospital's close by, but we still always argue about the way to get there. I think Paul goes the long way.

Even though I was only 28 when I had Nicola, my body was really feeling the strain and heaviness of pregnancy. The pain in my back was really bad and my legs were becoming more and more tired. And my body didn't bounce back the way it did when I was younger.

All the births since Robert were quite similar. I was always out of the hospital a day after each one and a midwife would come and check on us at home. But everything changed after Nicola.

By the time I was 29 and found out I was pregnant with our fifth child, I didn't have the insecurities I'd had with my first pregnancies. I still wasn't great with the medical profession—I'm the same with going to the dentist—but I was happy to have shared care once again.

This fifth pregnancy was absolutely fine and everything went really smoothly. Then, on 30 April 1999, when I was 37 weeks pregnant, I started to get some terrible back pain, which was much worse than anything I'd had so far during the pregnancy. That had always been the first sign of labour for me, so at about 7.30 that evening I got in the bath to try to relax.

But as soon as I got in, my waters broke and I panicked. That had never happened before and as I clambered out of the bath I yelled out to Paul, who was downstairs watching *Gardening Australia*. 'Ring the midwives,' I shouted. 'Ring the hospital. Find out what's happening.'

Nicola, who was just three, was asleep on the couch. Paul rang the hospital. 'She wants to know how many contractions you've had,' he yelled up. 'I haven't had any yet,' I shouted back.

I put on some exercise tights and a top and walked down the stairs to take the phone from Paul. And while I was explaining to the midwife that I hadn't had any contractions, one came and I let out a groan. 'Right,' she said. 'Get in the car. You need to come in straight away.'

I hung up and tried to bundle up the kids. 'Get in the car, get in the car,' I said as calmly as possible. Our eldest son Robert just took off and Paul started running in and out of the house. He got Michael and Kayler in the car but when he came back in to pick up Nicky, I could feel the baby move into the birth canal. 'I'm not going to make it!' I shouted. 'I'm not going to make it!'

I crossed my legs and stood at the doorway and thought, *No, this is not happening*, and Paul started dragging the kids back out of the car. 'Get off the tiles!' Paul shouted from the car—he thought the baby was just going to drop out onto the tiles. As I moved back towards the lounge room, a second contraction came.

I was just terrified. I was worried for the baby as it was two and a half weeks early and I was also concerned for Nicky, who'd just woken up and was freaking out on the couch. I went very quiet and thought, *Paul, where are you?*—and as I stood at the door of the lounge room, the baby just popped out. I pulled down my tights with one hand and grabbed hold of him with the other. There was no pushing—that second contraction did it all—and poor Nicola saw her baby brother being born.

My neighbour arrived—that's where Robert had gone—and she pulled out a dining room chair for me and I sat down with my newborn baby in my hands. It really was like something out of a rice field.

The baby made one little cry and while he looked healthy and his initial colour was good, I could tell he was rapidly losing body heat. I had started shaking uncontrollably—I went straight into shock—but I quickly snapped back into reality and somehow took control of the situation. 'We've got to keep the baby warm, we need to get him warm,' I said repeatedly. 'This is not good. Get some towels. Call an ambulance.'

There had been no tearing and there was hardly any mess, yet I felt such a mix of emotions. I was frightened but there was all this love and concern for both the baby, who we named Joshua, and Nicola. As I sat there in a daze, I almost felt like everyone was more concerned about getting the children out of the road than about Josh and me. Kayler came and cuddled Nicola, who was still in a state of shock, and the kids eventually went next door to the neighbours. Paul was on the phone trying to get hold of anybody to come. 'What are they doing, out shopping or something?' he kept saying.

I was starting to panic as the baby started to feel really cold—all my other babies were just so warm when they came out. The umbilical cord wasn't very long and I was also worried because we didn't have any clean scissors to cut it. But the ambulance came really quickly and someone soon put a blanket around me, cut the cord and took charge of the baby. The ambulance trolley couldn't get up to the landing, which had a little turn and a few more steps, so I had to walk to the ambulance with the cord hanging out of me and the placenta still inside. It wasn't a good look for the neighbours.

Joshua did get cold—all that coming and going at the front door meant that the cool night air had gotten into the house—and he had to spend eight hours warming up in a humidicrib. And poor little Nicky had been given such a fright. She didn't want to stay at the neighbours' that night so after coming to the hospital, Paul went home and got her. But the next day she was fine. 'Oh, this is my little baby,' she said when she came in to visit and she still teases Josh that she saw him being born, even though she can't really remember it.

I'd actually considered having a home birth with Joshua, but I'd always imagined it to be a lot more planned and relaxed and with a midwife there. But Paul had been against the idea. All my babies seemed to face the wrong way and he was concerned there might be complications because of that and wanted the safety of the hospital.

The shock of Joshua's birth didn't put me off having another baby, although I was a bit worried as the gestation period seemed to be getting shorter and shorter with each one. We were already up to two and a half weeks early and I was really concerned if we had another one it would be even earlier, which wouldn't be very good for the baby. So when I found out I was pregnant with our sixth child, I was immediately concerned. I was also concerned about my own health—eight months into the pregnancy with Josh, I could hardly walk and had to be rolled out of bed because of the pain in my back.

But the pregnancy was very normal. I went to the midwives' clinic and told them how concerned I was about having another quick birth and they talked about organising a midwife to be on call in the area before the due date, just in case. But that didn't quite eventuate.

I had my usual back pain towards the end of the pregnancy, and when I was 35 weeks I felt like I was coming down with a virus. It was 4 June 2002 and I'd felt sicky and nauseous all day and had a killer of a back pain all over. Everything just felt wrong, and I became worried when I didn't feel any better by about six o'clock that night. *I'm not having this kid here*, I thought.

'I don't feel well,' I said to Kayler, who was then 12 years old. 'I think I'll go into hospital.' 'Are you going to have the baby?' she asked. 'No,' I said. 'It's too early for that. I just don't feel right.'

We'd moved house by then and Paul was watching the European soccer on the TV downstairs, so I went up to the bedroom, but the pain in my back just got worse and worse. I picked up my bag and moved down to the kitchen, which was the central place in the house. I also knew it had a gas heater in there. 'Tell Dad we've got to go to the hospital right now,' I said to Kayler. And he just said to her, 'Tell Mum to wait until half-time.'

'No,' I said—it was too late. I couldn't wait. There'd been no warning: no show, no contraction, no waters breaking, no pushing, nothing—and all of a sudden the waters broke and the baby came with them. And there was Samuel in the kitchen and his older sister caught him.

Kayler was terrified, but she was so level-headed. She yelled out to Paul and started throwing towels into the dryer, boiling water and getting scissors and dental thread to tie the umbilical cord while I just stood there with the baby in my arms. She was very organised and did everything, while Paul didn't know whether he was coming or going. He took his jumper off, put it back on—and then took it off again. He was really caught on the hop.

It was such a fright but because of our experience with Josh, we knew what we were doing this time. My mind started racing ahead, thinking about how we needed to get this baby to the hospital and someone organised to look after the other five kids, but I felt like my body was acting so slowly. It was like I was in two dimensions.

Paul mopped the floor and my girlfriend arrived to look after the kids. And we decided that we could probably be at the hospital by the time the ambulance got there, so we cut the umbilical cord ourselves, wrapped up the baby and went to the hospital. They knew we were coming and although Samuel was early, and quite small, he was very healthy and he was back home in three days. He didn't get cold like Josh did.

My last two birth experiences were unconventional and pain free, but they were both a bit scary and weren't very comfortable. Both times I started shivering and shaking uncontrollably with my teeth chattering, and I just couldn't stop. It was annoying as I felt like I'd lost control again but it was just my body's way of saying, 'I'm coping, but you didn't give me time to ease into this.'

It took a while to physically recover from the last two births and emotionally I almost felt like I'd failed. I didn't give birth in a clinical, traditional environment and even though I'd had all those children, anything could have happened. I'm not a medical person and what if there was some little sign that something was wrong? Would I have picked that up? I felt a little guilty and probably would have felt it was my fault if things had gone wrong because I hadn't reacted in time. So although Samuel's and Joshua's births were wonderful in many ways, I had a lot of self-doubt about them. But really, it was just a relief to see the babies safe and alert.

I'd never say no to more children but I don't think my body would like to have any more. My back has really gone, I have terrible varicose veins that haven't shrunk back and it really took my body longer to recover after each birth. I actually felt depressed after Samuel's birth. I felt my body had failed me and I cried and cried thinking I couldn't do it any more. But I suppose if it came to crunch time, I'd probably go on a health kick and go through it again, but I would be very paranoid in that last trimester, thinking the baby would come way too early.

We used to get stacks of people saying, 'You're young parents.' Now they say, 'Look at all these children', so you can't really win. But it's been very natural for us. It's always nice to have a baby around the house and Paul and I always wanted a big family, probably to replace the love we feel we may have missed out on from our own families. The children have their moments, but they all look after each other. Hopefully, we're giving them a wonderful life and they'll appreciate us and each other, although I'm sure our 16 year old would have been quite happy if we'd stopped at two. Then he could have had his own room.

Postscript

Not content with the handful that goes with having six children, Jane Torley and her bookkeeper husband, Paul, home-school Kayler, Michael and Nicola. 'Michael was not coping in a normal school, so we decided to home-school him,' says Jane 35. 'And then when we did one, we thought we might as well do the younger ones as well.'

The main reason the couple chose to teach their own children was to make sure that none of them got lost in the education system. 'It's a reassuring thing,' she says of the routine they review every three months. 'I wanted to protect them and I didn't want anyone to slip down anywhere.'

While she admits she is 'more protective than she used to be', Jane says her family, which lives in Canberra, is very different to the one she grew up in. 'We talk about so many different issues that we would never have discussed in my home growing up,' she says. 'Everything's very open. If anyone has a question they can come to us. Sometimes it can be in the middle of dinner and they may ask some terrible question and you think, "Couldn't that have waited until later?" But at least it's dealt with and everything's light-hearted.'

She says she chooses not to think about the traumatic time surrounding the birth of her first child, but knows it's an experience her daughters will never have to go through. 'If they were in a similar situation,' she says, 'I would totally prepare them for it.'

The only time Jane gets to herself is at 'two in the morning', she jokes, but it's obvious she wouldn't have it any other way and looks forward to even more children overrunning the house. 'My grandmother had a lot of children and we'd always go home to Grandma's and all the relatives would be there,' says Jane, who still manages to work part-time in floristry. 'I'd like to think that we'd be the new grandma's house one day.'

Completing the jigsaw

LINDA BURNEY

I was born in 1957 in Whitton, a tiny country town in the Riverina, in south-western New South Wales. My mother was 20, white and unmarried. I was black.

I don't know too many details but I do know it was an absolute scandal. My mother left the hospital where I was born before I did and it was her aunt and uncle, two non-Aboriginal people who were brother and sister, unmarried and in their mid to late sixties, who took me home and raised me. My grandmother lived next door, so I saw my mother when she visited, but if it weren't for my Aunt Nina and Uncle Billy I would probably have ended up becoming lost in the system, being fostered out somewhere.

We were dirt poor. I used to go and collect wood on a horse and dray with my uncle and I had a real country kid's life, riding horses, swimming in the irrigation channels, making forts in the bush. Aunt Nina and Uncle Billy were really frugal people and gave me great groundings in life—

the importance of honesty, loyalty and treating people well.

I had a loving upbringing and never felt rejected by any stretch, but I didn't have a close relationship with my mother. And I didn't know who my father was. My heritage was never discussed. It was just so taboo, a complete shame.

I probably became aware that I was different from my cousins when I was about six years old. I saw a photograph a travelling photographer had taken, and there they all were, white, blond and blue-eyed, and there was me, this really little dark kid on the end. But it wasn't until I was about 13 that it became a serious issue of identity for me.

It was around this time that I sat alone on the front verandah of our home and literally pictured a road with a fork in it. I thought, *Well, I can take one fork and pretend I am Maori or Spanish.* Some people used to do that as a way of surviving, which would have been a terrible lie of denial. *Or I can take the path of who and what I am.* And that's what I decided to do. But it was of my own volition and I had to figure it all out by myself, so although I had a good childhood, there was always this really sad, uncompleted part of me which was very private.

After Aunt Nina and Uncle Billy died, I lived with my best girlfriend's incredibly generous family so I could finish Year 10 at Leeton High School and then moved to Penrith to live with my mother and stepfather for the first time, and did the HSC. I was 17 and my relationship with my mother never developed. She died two years later in 1976 when I was studying to be a teacher in Bathurst and she'd never told me who my father was. It just wasn't a conversation we had.

I spent my early to mid twenties working as a teacher,

becoming active in Aboriginal education and activist roles, and looking for my father. As an Aboriginal person, knowing where your country is and who your relations are is fundamental to who you are, and I really needed to know where I was from. And my father was the key.

I had no idea where to start looking—he could have been anywhere—but I concentrated my efforts on Whitton and Leeton. I asked questions and wrote letters to people who had known me all my life, the doctor who delivered me and also the midwife, and nobody seemed to know anything. And I faced a lot of ignorance and racism throughout it all. One of the older non-Aboriginal women in the town, who knew me really well, actually said, 'You're doing so well, why do you need to know that?'

I also put it out amongst the community that I was trying to find my heritage. The Aboriginal grapevine works in spectacular ways and eventually I started to hear little things. Soon, someone mentioned that one of the girls I went to high school with was my cousin. So I started to get to know some of the people around the community in Leeton and I felt I was getting closer.

I wasn't thinking at all about having my own children at the time. I had extraordinarily irregular periods and the doctors had told me there was probably a real chance that I wasn't going to be able to fall pregnant. In the back of my mind, I knew I probably could because I'd had a termination when I was about 18. But I really didn't have any expectations as I only had one or two periods a year and hadn't been using contraception for seven years. So I was really shocked when I found out at 27 that I was pregnant with my first child. I was four months on before

I realised. The pregnancy was unplanned, but not unwanted.

It was a relatively easy pregnancy physically although there were some very stressful moments. I was living in this little, tiny, old terrace in Erskineville with my partner at the time, Chris, and a very close friend, Michael. Living in an Aboriginal household, you've got people in and out all the time and I had all of that which was great.

I was working in a really important job as head of the NSW Aboriginal Education Consultancy Group, so I didn't have time to think too much about the pregnancy, although everyone else around me did. There were lots of old aunties and uncles and many friends throughout the community who were really looking forward to the baby arriving.

I didn't do the whole antenatal trip and I hadn't really thought about the birth. I saw the doctors as minimally as I needed to. I knew that you had to breathe slowly and that was about it.

I didn't have romantic ideas about it. My view was that in Western society it's as if you're the only woman who's ever had a baby when you become pregnant. But birth happens millions of times every day—it's just a part of life, like death. And even though it might be painful, it's just 24 hours, one day of your life, where it's going to be uncomfortable for a wonderful outcome. I also thought about women back in the industrial revolution who went and had their babies and were back on the production line straight away. I had a really intellectual view about how I was going to get through the whole thing, which was probably a blessing.

Then, on 18 April 1984, when I was eight months'

pregnant, I was sitting at home and my friend Maureen came around unexpectedly. 'I've got someone for you to meet,' she said simply. 'I think we've found your father.' I found a photo of my mother at the age he would have known her, put on some shoes and went with her.

She drove me down to a conference centre in Coogee near the beach and as I sat in the back of the car, I saw this stunningly handsome man walk across the road. He was wearing a blue shirt, a black cowboy hat and had really dark brown, beautiful eyes.

He got in the car and I asked, 'Do you know a woman called Rita Burney?' which was my mother's name. 'No, I don't,' he replied. I showed him the photograph and again he said, 'I don't know her.' And my whole world just fell away.

And then suddenly, after nearly a minute's silence, something just clicked. And he put his arms around me and said, 'I hope I don't disappoint you.'

It was beyond description. Here was my father, Noni. I could see how I looked like him—he had the same huge smile as mine—but I didn't know him. And the fact that I was meeting him for the first time and was pregnant out to there was incredible.

He was returning to Narrandera that night, so Maureen drove us out to the airport and we had a couple of hours together. He told me a bit about where he came from and about the family's history. It turned out I'd actually grown up in my country and he, and my ten brothers and sisters, lived only 40 minutes' drive away. I guess I felt a little cheated, but most of all I was in shock from the enormity of it all.

And there was this incredible sunset while we sat at the airport. And at the same time Chris, who was in Collarenebri, eight or nine hours' drive away, had stopped on the road because the sunset was so amazing.

It was quite hard to make small talk for the entire time we were together but Noni was incredibly proud of me. And when he left, we knew there were a lot more things to say and people to meet, but I also felt I wasn't going to push myself on to this man. I would just let things take their natural course.

Maureen drove me home and I spent the evening on my own, stunned, but just so relieved. Then, at two o'clock in the morning, my membranes came away and I went into early labour. The emotion of meeting my dad had caused it all to happen four weeks' early.

Michael, my great friend, and his brother were staying at the house, so I went and woke them up. 'Um, the baby's coming,' I said. They got up quickly, but it was hilarious. They were sitting there drinking tea and smoking cigarettes in a complete flap, saying, 'Well, hurry up, Linda.' And there I was making them cups of tea between spasms and trying to iron something reasonable to wear to the hospital.

I was completely unprepared. I didn't even have a nightgown. There was no bassinette, nothing like that. And I was actually booked in for my first antenatal class at 7.30 the next evening.

For the first half hour or so the pain seemed bearable. We weren't timing the contractions—there was nothing scientific about it—but I knew I wanted to get to the hospital. So Michael drove me up at about five o'clock in the morning.

Word seemed to spread very quickly, and early in the piece one of my friends came in and ran down to Grace Bros to get me something to wear. My girlfriends did shifts and someone was with me the whole time while Christopher drove back from Collarenebri.

It was an amazing day. So many people came up to the hospital and the mood was actually quite festive early on. I was head of an Aboriginal organisation, it was my first baby and it was big news. There were people on the balcony peeking into the delivery room when the nurse was out. There were people ringing all the time and the hospital absolutely got the shits. They actually came in and asked me if I could do something about the amount of people calling up. But all these people were really dear friends who were just so excited for me.

The pain was in waves and after a while it became really exhausting. The contractions weren't ten or fifteen minutes' apart. Right from the word go, they were every few minutes. And I just wasn't dilating.

Eventually, the midwives put some gel on my cervix, which didn't seem to help, and they also gave me some sort of injection. Soon, I became just so tired, stressed and distressed and it wasn't much fun at all. I was an absolute physical wreck.

Chris arrived—he had plenty of time to drive back— and after about 14 hours of labour I had an epidural. I was not into natural childbirth or anything like that. I was so tired and over it that it was just another procedure.

But it went wrong. I'm so tiny and they had enormous difficulty trying to find the space between the vertebrae to do it. They poked and prodded for a long time before they found a space and then they stuffed it up—it pierced the spinal cord and my spinal fluid leaked out. I was in agony. It was all right when I was lying flat, but when I sat up it was just torture. My head felt like it was going to come off my shoulders.

There was also a monitor on me because I'd been in labour for so long and the baby was starting to show signs of distress. And when it finally got to the point of delivery and they'd been trying and trying and trying, the doctor, who was now using forceps, said, 'If you don't deliver this time, it's going to be a Caesarean.' And I did deliver that time—after 27 hours of labour—but I had an enormous amount of internal and external stitches.

They put him on me and I felt really happy, but I was just so exhausted. And his father cried. I wouldn't say it was a beautiful moment, but it was a great moment of relief. He was this tiny five-pound thing, so thin and little. He reminded me of a beautiful little frog. And he was all bruised and scraped up. He also had a birthmark on his left eyelid and black curly hair.

We named him Binni Dironbirong, which came from the meeting I had with my father. Binni is the strength and shaft of a spear and Dironbirong is the red colours of the setting sun. His birth symbolises to us the fact he was born when I met the Aboriginal side of my family.

I didn't really feel the pain of the botched epidural during the birth—there was too much else going on—but once I went back to my room I couldn't sit up. I had to lie flat. So even after the birth I was in pain. There was so much intervention.

The anaesthetist came back to patch up my spinal cord

two or three days later, which meant I had to have another epidural. You can put up with the epidural when you're in agony but getting one when you're not in childbirth isn't fun.

It wasn't a textbook delivery. Binni was so little and not well. He had really bad jaundice, which made it difficult for him to feed, and he was in a humidicrib for a long time, longer than I needed to stay in hospital. I ended up staying for ten days, partly because I was pretty knocked around but also because he was not ready to feed properly and come home. 'Stay in there as long as you can,' a friend of mine said, 'because it's the last rest you're going to get.' Binni stayed in hospital an extra few days and I used to go up and feed him.

I turned 28 when I was in hospital—there were so many flowers and gifts—and when I brought Binni home his first bed was a drawer, and a couple of girlfriends had cleaned the house for me, which was lovely.

My second pregnancy was also a great shock. If anyone ever says breastfeeding's a great method of contraception, it's rubbish. I discovered five months after giving birth to Binni that I was pregnant again.

The second pregnancy might have also been unplanned, but it was a dream. I can't remember losing any energy and I kept working in a really high-profile job, right up to the week before I had the baby.

I started having contractions while I was shopping with a friend at the old Grace Bros building in Broadway, Sydney, in the early evening of 22 August 1986. We finished buying whatever we were buying, but I couldn't drive. We got home, got Chris out of a meeting and at about 20 to seven, he raced me up to the hospital. He let me out of the car, they put me in a wheelchair and took me to the delivery room. Chris parked the car and just as he came into the room I was giving birth.

I didn't need any assistance. There was no drama or drugs and solid labour was about 20 minutes. After our little girl was born, I got off the bed, put on a pair of jeans—my body went straight back to thin—and went to the public phone and started ringing people to tell them I'd had a baby girl. I'd seen some of them that afternoon and they all said, 'What? Unbelievable.' And Chris was home in time to watch the football that night, which he was very pleased about.

She was small, six pounds, but not as tiny as her brother. And she was beautiful. She reminded me of a perfect almond. She was a glowing brown colour and had these enormous dark, oriental-shaped eyes with eyelashes that touched her eyebrows. There was not a mark on her. She wasn't wrinkly or scaly. She was like a little doll.

There was a huge rainstorm when I had Willurai, and that's the overwhelming thing that I recall from her birth—not the speed of it, not the pain. It was just that I could hear it raining heavily. Her name is Willurai Ngurumbi Karamarra. Willurai means bush honey, that sweet sap that comes out of a particular tree, Ngurumbi means winter—she was born in August—and Karamarra means water.

Both the children were named as a result of the circumstances surrounding their births. Their father is interested in linguistics and we had the Wiradjuri language dictionary. The irony is that two Aboriginal people had to go back to a dictionary, but it's a nice way of reclaiming the language and it means a lot to the kids and their identity. And no matter where I am in the world, when I look at a pink or red sunset I think of that moment, of my son, and when it rains heavily I think of Willurai.

The births were two completely different experiences, and I sometimes wonder if the nature of a child's birth and pregnancy shapes the child. Binni came into this world in really tough circumstances and he wears life heavily at times, whereas, in some ways Willurai's more easygoing.

I also believe the way your children are born determines a great deal about how you treat and relate to them for the rest of their lives. I'm much more protective and perhaps a bit softer with Binni than I am with his sister because his start was so difficult and hers wasn't. I'm not sure how fair that is, but it's probably just an unconscious thing we do.

Becoming a mother was a real challenge for me because I wasn't sure what mothering was all about. I had a loving upbringing but never a mother. I've always wanted to give my children everything I missed out on and I hope it hasn't affected my capacity to be a loving parent.

The thing I did take from the very beginning was that I could combine work and being a mother. My kids went into childcare when they were a few months old and I didn't see them as an interruption to my career. I never thought I had to stop work to be a good mother. And being a stay-at-home mum didn't sit well with me—I felt like my brain was turning into a giant cabbage by the time Binni was about three or four months old.

Chris and I separated about three years after Willurai was born, so I was a single mum for a lot of the time when she and Binni were little. I made an enormous effort to read with them at night, and tried to get to all their school things.

But Aboriginal children sacrifice a lot if their mother or father's involved in the struggle. As a parent, you're constantly, sometimes unsuccessfully, finding the balance between your responsibilities and the greater good.

Yet what is fantastic about being an Aboriginal person and in a community organisation is that my children have this enormous network of aunties and uncles. In our community, if someone is older and a friend of your mum's, you're required to call them auntie or uncle even though they might not be related.

Lots of people share ownership of children in Aboriginal communities—when you have a baby, he or she is not just yours, they're passed around to everyone and there really is a broad support system. I've got photos of Willo being breastfed at a protest in the Domain, and one of the wonderful presents Binni was given when he was born was a little red, black and yellow hand-knitted jumpsuit with the Aboriginal flag on it, which he wore to his first rally. They've been going to rallies and protests and meetings and on planes since they were tiny and have this fantastic extended communal family which is just wonderful.

It gave me a great deal of peace meeting my father before Binni was born. It meant my children would grow up knowing where they fitted into the Aboriginal kinship and cultural system, which is really important. They weren't going to grow up with the dilemma and sadness I grew up with and feeling like a half-finished jigsaw. They would always know exactly where they were from.

Postscript

In 2003, Burney became the first Aboriginal Parliamentarian for New South Wales and is now the Labor member for the western Sydney suburb of Canterbury. She lives in Marrickville with her partner since 1997, former National Farmers' Federation executive director Rick Farley, while her teenage children live with their father in the next suburb. 'It's quite a flexible arrangement and works really well,' she says. 'After growing up not knowing my father, I was really determined that the children had a great relationship with their dad and they do.'

During the past five years, Burney and Farley, who has two children from a previous marriage, have lost two pregnancies. One was a boy, close to five months. 'We desperately wanted a child,' she says. 'The sadness with losing both, particularly the pregnancy that got so far, is really burnt into me, and I know it is in Rick too. I still think of it regularly, even though it happened three years ago.'

Burney says that even though the couple may not have their own young child, 'we have lots of gorgeous children around us, that love us and we can give to'. And besides, she says with a smile, 'I'll probably have my own grandkids soon.'

The short distance between life and death

ANNE STANLEY

Darren and I met at high school in Mackay and started going out together when I was just 16. He was in his senior year and I was in Year 11. I was so young, but we both had a sense we were going to be together for a long time.

We were married in 1993 in Brisbane when I was 25 and after about five years of marriage we decided to start trying for children. I'd always imagined we'd have children and wanted to have a baby by the time I was 30.

We tried for about a year, but nothing happened. I had a laparoscopy to check if there were any problems with my uterus and ovaries and, although I had a bit of endometriosis, everything else seemed fine. We moved to London in 1999 for Darren's work and continued to try, unsuccessfully, by ourselves. The doctors ended up calling it 'unexplained infertility'.

It was just so terrible. There wasn't a day I didn't think about it and there was a huge battle going on in my mind as I was trying to work out how I was going to live the rest of my life without children. And I couldn't talk to my husband about it after a while—I'd just dissolve into tears.

Eventually, after three years of no luck and some terribly dark times, we decided to seek help. Our attitude was, let's investigate every option and if it turns out we're never going to have children, then let's deal with it then.

The fertility clinic in London did a stream of tests and told us that if we continued to try ourselves, we'd have a 5 per cent chance of falling pregnant, and if we tried intra uterine insemination, we'd have a 16 per cent one. We had a 30 per cent chance if we tried IVF, so we decided to go with the option that gave us the best statistics.

It was a huge step to take. We had to admit that falling pregnant was probably not going to happen by itself and the only chance we had was by doing something as impersonal and invasive as IVF. But we felt positive once we'd made the commitment. We were moving forward and our brains just switched over to 'so this is the way we're going to have our children'. We were doing what we needed to start a family.

I had my eggs removed under a local and two embryos were transferred. They put a little catheter inside me and then sent them up. It was like having a Pap smear.

We had to wait two weeks to see if we were pregnant and when I did the test in our tiny little London bathroom, we couldn't look at first. But it was positive. We were so happy and I phoned some friends and howled to them down the line. It was wonderful to think that we were finally pregnant after all we'd been through.

I had an ultrasound at six weeks to see the heartbeat and it was beautiful. I felt this baby was incredibly precious—

selfishly, more precious than anyone else's pregnancy. But then, at eight weeks, I started bleeding. They scanned me again and they found a haematoma, a blood bubble, right next to the baby. 'We can't do anything about it,' the doctor said. 'It will either stay the same and not affect the baby or it could grow bigger and force the baby to be aborted. Or it could go away by itself.'

So not long after the biggest high of my life, we were on tenterhooks again. And then, one night during my eleventh week of pregnancy, I suddenly felt more bleeding. I went to the loo and it gushed out of me like a flood. It was my worst nightmare coming true.

I was hysterical. I phoned the IVF clinic immediately and they told us we had to wait until the morning to be scanned. 'Are you in any pain?' asked the person on the end of the line. I wasn't. 'Well, that's a good thing,' she said.

The next morning they had a look and there was the baby. It was actually the haematoma that was releasing the blood. I was so relieved and happy and from then on, the baby continued to grow and all its measurements showed it was a very big, healthy baby.

I had a very good pregnancy after that. I was really happy but quite anxious to do everything right. And I was checked constantly. As a friend of mine who went through IVF once said, 'You become very good friends with the vaginal probe.'

We'd planned to come home to Australia at around 22 weeks, but my doctor at the IVF clinic thought a long plane journey might cause premature labour after the earlier problems we'd had. And that put us in a complete spin. All our stuff was already packed on a ship home and

Darren had finished up work. And I really didn't want to have our first baby away from friends and family. But after consulting other specialists who thought it would be okay to fly, we made our journey home, albeit a little fearfully, and everything was fine.

We were very happy to be home and I started researching what birth would be like. Darren and I went to an active birth seminar, which encouraged women to move around during labour, and it was great. And I really enjoyed doing yoga. I felt that I was fairly empowered to manage the pain, but I had an open mind. I wanted to see how I went, but if the pain turned out to be more than I could bear I would go for the drugs.

I had a lot of Braxton Hicks contractions from week 20 and by the time my due date came around in late May 2001, I was already four centimetres dilated. I couldn't believe it and when I left my obstetrician's office I was convinced the baby would come that night. But it didn't.

Eight days later I went back to my obstetrician and although I had dilated another centimetre, she suggested an induction, which I wasn't very keen about. I really wanted everything to be as natural as possible and I'd heard scary stories about inductions being so monumental. But our overwhelming feeling was concern for the baby. We were too anxious to let it go any longer.

I checked into the hospital the following morning and at 8 a.m. my doctor broke my waters and an hour later I had the syntocinon drip plugged into my arm. The pains came instantly. My adrenalin was racing and I had to focus on breathing through the contractions straight away. But it was manageable and I wasn't frightened by it.

I was on my feet the whole time. Darren stood behind me and put his hand on the middle of my forehead—the third eye in yoga—and I just swayed and breathed through the pain. It was all a bit herbally and I'm not really a herbally kind of person, but in this case I was quite happy to try it and it seemed to work.

The contractions were thick and fast—half a minute apart at most—and the midwife suggested I try different positions. But whenever I moved I regretted it because I felt I'd lost control. I'd become fixated on two things—the warmth of Darren's hand and the warm spot on the metal trolley that had the drip attached to it—and I knew I could manage the pain if I could feel both those things.

After two hours of labour, the midwife checked my cervix and I was nine centimetres dilated. I knew I wasn't going to be able to move again after climbing onto that bed, so the gas became my next focus point. And as I breathed out I made a noise, just like in yoga, to get rid of tension. I probably sounded like a cow, mooing down into that mask.

The intensity of the contractions seemed to increase and it soon came to the point where I could have used more serious pain relief, but my midwife told me they'd phoned my doctor and she would be here in 40 minutes. I decided I could manage for that long and continued groaning at the top of my voice through the gas pipe.

And then everything went a bit panicked and a midwife whipped an oxygen mask on to my face. 'I'm just going to put this on,' she said. 'Everything's all right. Your baby's getting the oxygen you're breathing.'

I had a monitor on my tummy and there was obviously something wrong with the baby's heartbeat. But I was removed from it all—I was in so much pain and was just trying to manage that. Later I found out the baby had been in foetal distress.

The midwives kept telling me my doctor was coming, but they flipped me onto my side and a horrid midwife shoved her hand up inside me without telling me what she was doing. It was excruciating—I certainly sounded like a cow then—but I later found out she was trying to clear the cord around the baby's head.

My obstetrician soon arrived and said the baby needed to come out straight away, so she put my legs in lithotomy stirrups and put a ventouse cap in—the second most painful moment of the whole thing. I pushed while she pulled. 'You've got to do the biggest poo you've ever done,' she said. Initially, I was trying to push out from my vagina, but I really had to push out of my rectum, and I was convinced every vein in my backside was going to burst.

The baby's head was delivered after 20 minutes of pushing. It was such a relief—but it was incredibly hard to summon up the energy to deliver the rest. And then, suddenly there was this huge baby boy. They put him on my tummy and I was absolutely amazed by his strength and how big and powerful he was. He was a huge life-force, all four kilos of him.

And I tore—right up to my rectum. I had told my husband before the birth that I really didn't want stitches and here I was with a secondary tear. 'It's not muscle,' my doctor said. 'It's only skin.'

The stitching was horrible. All I wanted to do was close

my legs and relax for a moment and I was left cringing at every feeling from then on. She said that in six weeks I wouldn't know she'd been there, which wasn't strictly true.

Apart from the stitches I really enjoyed giving birth to Patrick and I don't think his birth could have been better. I felt I'd worked hard and produced something amazing. And to go through that pain was a learning experience for me. I got through it and I managed it.

We decided to try for another child when Patrick was about 18 months old. I was 35 and we thought it might take a few years for us to be successful again on IVF. But it was a totally different experience this time. We didn't have the anxieties and stresses of the first time. We were much more positive and I was impatient—I just wanted to get through the process to see what would happen at the other end.

But I always felt guilty going to the IVF clinic. There were all these people in the waiting room who might have been trying over and over for children and there we were with this beautiful little blond toddler, zooming around and being as cute as a button. We felt like we were being greedy. But we really wanted another child.

When we found out we were pregnant again after our first transfer, we couldn't believe our luck. And to our delight, we saw two little hearts beating at our first ultrasound.

It was as if we'd won the lottery. Only two years earlier, I was trying to get used to the idea that I might never have children. And here I was, soon to have three children under three, Patrick and two babies, who we later found out were girls.

We were ecstatic, but we were also concerned that having twins meant the pregnancy would be risky. And it wasn't too long before I got quite bad morning sickness, which made it hard to cope with a little toddler.

My IVF doctor told me he didn't think an obstetrician would deliver twins vaginally. But my obstetrician, a different one to the one who delivered Patrick, was full of optimism. 'Oh no, I always deliver my twins normally,' she said. 'You'll be fine. You had a really good birth with Patrick and these babies will be a breeze. We'll deliver the first one and then if the other one's head isn't down, I'll try and turn her around. And if I can't, I'll go in there and pull her out.' I felt really comfortable and confident with her approach and I really couldn't see a reason to have abdominal surgery if I didn't need to.

By about 29 weeks, I was fairly big and very uncomfortable with back pain, but I was convinced I was going to go a long way with these twins, so Darren and I decided to take Patrick on a little farm-stay holiday. We went out for dinner to the local pub on the Saturday night and while we were there, I felt some bleeding. I rang the hospital, which was only an hour's drive away, and they told me to come in.

I was pretty relaxed because it was only a small amount, but after an examination they wouldn't let me go home. I was scanned the next day and it showed that my cervix had started to thin. And my doctor decided I needed to stay. 'If you go home, you'll be on your feet even if you say you'll lie down,' she said. 'We've got to get these babies as big as possible.' So I had to remain in hospital, on complete bed rest, until the babies came.

I was devastated. I didn't know what we were going to do and how we were going to manage with Patrick. And we hadn't prepared a thing for the girls. I was also miserable because I had to lie in one position. And that was painful, especially as I got bigger.

Mum came down from Mackay and, thankfully, took charge at home. I missed Patrick terribly, but I never really worried about the health of the babies. All the scans showed they were a good size for their age and the doctors gave me steroid shots to help develop their lungs. I always felt they would be okay.

But I was concerned about the way they were going to begin their lives. I knew they would have to be put straight into isolette boxes to keep them warm and that I wouldn't be able to hold them and they'd be fed through tubes. And I also knew I'd probably have to go home without them and that was awful to think about.

After a couple of miserable weeks in hospital, I started having contractions which would wake me up during the night. And then, at 31 weeks and five days my waters broke while I was sitting up in bed, having lunch. The nurse took me down to the labour room and I rang Darren, who rushed over from work.

I really didn't want to have an epidural, but my doctor said it was a good idea in case she had to turn the second baby around. So the anaesthetist was sent down to give me an epidural and it was awful. It was like cold metal running down my spine. I also didn't like having to lie on the bed with all these bits attached to me, but I knew it was necessary.

It was strange having the epidural when I wasn't in any pain. It was a good one though, as I could feel some pain when the contractions peaked. I didn't want to feel removed from the whole process. But I could still keep on chatting and blissfully let it all happen.

The contractions came on strongly throughout the afternoon and by about six o'clock, my obstetrician arrived and checked my cervix. I was nine centimetres dilated. She told me I didn't need to be fully dilated because the babies were small, and I definitely felt the urge to push, so she put me into the lithotomy position, sitting up in bed with my legs up in the air in stirrups once again.

I asked for a mirror to watch as I pushed the baby out and I found that really motivating. Darren, however, was not so keen. Later on he told me he would have preferred not to have seen that part of the birth.

After about seven big pushes, Olivia was delivered. They put her cheek to my cheek and I was so surprised by how full of life she was. I thought she would be puny and weak and frightening-looking. But she wasn't. She was just a small, healthy baby, howling and kicking her legs, in the same way Patrick had, even though she was just 1.9 kilos.

They whisked her away to be rugged up and checked by the paediatrician and our thinking switched instantly to the second baby. She was still lying cross-wise, so my doctor moved herself into position on a little stool between my legs and started pushing the top of my stomach to try and flip her round. But it didn't work.

After a little while, she said, 'I'm going to have to go in and get her out.' But there was no real concern in her voice—and just as she reached inside to break my waters, they gushed out in three huge whooshes, like a fire hydrant. It was bizarre. She jumped back and shrieked and got absolutely drenched from her stomach to her toes and we all had a laugh.

She sat down again and then went in to try and grab the baby's feet. It was like something from *All Creatures Great and Small*—she was up to her elbow, digging around, and even though I could feel her hand moving, there was no pain at all thanks to the epidural. 'Now there's the foot,' she said, her eyes fixed off into the distance. 'No, I can't get it. I can't get it. That's the hand, no, I've got a foot.'

I was staring intently at her face and could sense she was getting agitated, when suddenly she stopped and pulled her arm out. 'No,' she said. 'This is no good. This baby's not coming. We've got to get this baby out right now.' And as she quickly pushed her chair back and headed for the door, she told the midwife, 'Whack that emergency button. Let's get people running around here.'

I was all strapped up to a monitor and the baby's heartbeat had dropped right down. And as the nurse hit the button, people started pulling off leads while others tried to re-attach bits of the bed and find something to cover me. All I could think was, *Just wheel me down like this. I don't care if I haven't got a blanket over my legs, just go!* I was gripped by fear and panic and started shaking uncontrollably.

Darren began running around the room ripping plugs out of the walls, and as they wheeled me down to the delivery theatre I prayed out loud, 'God, please look after my baby.' I really feared I could wake up on the other side and my baby could be dead.

Darren and I didn't say a word to each other. He held my hand as he ran alongside me down the hallway about four doors away and as they pushed me through the theatre doors I could see people dressed in gowns and I saw them hold Darren back.

I still had the umbilical cord hanging out of me from Olivia's birth and they tried to lift me onto the operating table but I couldn't move. They went to put the mask over my face and I said, 'Please, can somebody stay with my husband.' They said, 'Yes, someone will be with him.' And then I blacked out.

I woke up crying after the operation with Darren and my obstetrician by my side. As I bawled uncontrollably, she stroked my hand and face and told me that she had delivered the baby but it had been very difficult to get her out. My uterus had clamped down like a rubber band, halfway up around the baby, so it was trapped in the top of my uterus. She told me she couldn't pull her out of the normal Caesarean cut and was only moments away from doing a vertical Caesarean when she managed to get her out. She'd never had this happen throughout her 20 years of delivering babies. A few days later she talked to me about the shock—for both of us—of realising what a short difference it was between life and death. If it had taken any longer for them to get the baby out, anything could have happened.

I was in a daze and couldn't stop crying. They wheeled me on my bed into the nursery to see the babies and they were in their isolette boxes with oxygen apparatus over their faces and cords and wires stuck to them. They had little white paper, sunglass-shaped bandages around their heads and the one who'd been born by Caesarean, who we'd named Laura, was very badly bruised. It was as if her feet had been dipped in dark purple ink.

As I lay there, I felt quite removed, particularly from Laura. It was the first time I'd seen her and I really couldn't see anything of her, just this little body with all the bits and pieces attached.

I returned to the ward and they told me the girls were doing fine and they gave me a little Polaroid shot of them which I held all night. I eventually stopped sobbing, but I was in shock. And I also had drips and cords attached to me from the Caesarean and I could hardly move.

Poor Darren had been given a terrible fright. In many ways the whole experience was a lot harder for him emotionally as he thought he might have lost me too. I know he felt quite helpless and I heard that when the people in the nursery offered him a drink, he'd told them, 'You don't have the kind of drink I really need.'

The whole thing seemed to have taken so long but somehow they managed to deliver the girls about 15 to 18 minutes apart. My obstetrician had previously told me that they didn't like to have the deliveries more than 20 minutes apart, so they really did an amazing job. We felt so lucky the babies were as healthy as they were and the next morning the paediatrician allayed any fears I had about Laura's birth or head trauma. He said she probably had more trauma to her limbs because she was delivered breech.

I felt so sad to not have been with Laura when she was born and still have some sadness about it. She didn't have anybody with her—neither Darren nor me—and was put straight into an isolette box. Anything could have happened to her.

The girls rallied quite quickly though. They were both off the oxygen by the next morning, but it was a struggle for them—and for me. I was trying to recover from the birth and also wanted to be there for the girls. I was in a lot of pain. I didn't sleep that first night and by the second night I was still sitting with them at nine o'clock, with my IV drip in, exhausted and unshowered. I felt awful for those first few days and didn't know what was expected of me. I often thought, *Would other mothers be down here? Should I be sitting beside them every moment?*

I was surprised I didn't recover from the Caesarean better than I did. Friends of mine had had Caesareans and were up walking around the next day. I could hardly move. I still couldn't get out of bed to go to the toilet without tears of pain several days later. I think the birth must have been quite brutal.

It was very strange not having the twins in my room. I couldn't just sit and watch them and cuddle them. We were able to put our hands in their little boxes and touch them and change their nappies, but the first time I nursed them was three days after they were born. That's a very long time and I really didn't feel anything for them in a way. The whole bonding thing took a long time and it was very different to our experience with Patrick. It was all so confusing. I left hospital nine days after the births, alone. It was horrible to leave them but I really wanted to go home. I was quite torn, because I also felt guilty about being happy at home in my own environment with Patrick. I was emotionally exhausted and it was all too much, so I just sat there and howled.

But it was incredibly special when I held Olivia and Laura together for the first time, two weeks after their births. I finally felt like I had twins. My arms were overflowing with babies and it just filled me up. And it was a joyous day when they finally came home after nearly seven weeks.

I do sometimes wonder if it would have been safer and easier on us all if I'd had an elective Caesarean once we knew we were having twins. It would have been calmer all round and probably an easier recovery. But I would have missed out on delivering Olivia and that was really special.

And the important thing is where we got to. I'm perfectly fine and the girls are perfectly fine. And really, with the twins and a toddler, my life is too busy to have the luxury of dwelling on whether I made the right choices. We keep on going and live for our future. Our lives have turned around and we just couldn't be more fortunate.

Postscript

Anne Stanley and her engineer husband Darren have well and truly bonded with their daughters, who have now caught up with their age. 'They're no longer like premmie babies,' says Anne, who lives with her family in Brisbane. 'They're doing everything they're supposed to do and they've really stacked on the weight.'

They've also developed their own personalities. 'Even though Laura had the more traumatic birth, she has a much calmer personality than Olivia,' says Anne. 'She's a very placid, easygoing, smiley baby who wakes up happily.'

They also look quite different—Laura has blonde curls stacked up on her head, while Olivia has straight hair that sticks up like a mohawk, which Anne describes as 'very 1980s new wave, very Thompson Twins'.

Both Anne and her husband are more than happy with their brood of three, but they have unintentionally found themselves in a fertility dilemma. They recently received a bill from Monash IVF in Brisbane, charging them to store an unused frozen embryo, and they will one day have to decide whether to keep or destroy it. 'It's an ethical, moral thing that I can't quite get my head around,' says Anne. 'I definitely do not want to go through another pregnancy or birth again, but I just don't know if I could make the decision to destroy it. I think about this little frozen embryo. This potential fourth child could be something totally amazing.'

While her battle-weary husband initially couldn't believe she was even suggesting having another baby, Anne says he later came to understand her quandary. They have since paid for another six months of storage.

'I felt like a she-wolf who'd gone to the hills'

NIKKI GEMMELL

I used to tell my girlfriends at school that I didn't want children. I was going to be the cool one who'd be more interested in a career. In my twenties, it looked like it was going to be that way. I was completely focused on writing short stories whenever I could, and on my career as a journalist. The last thing I wanted was the pram in the hallway.

But something changed for me in my late twenties. My periods started getting heavier and more painful and suddenly I had this deep physical urge. Little triggers in my body were telling me it was time to have a baby. It was such an unexpected biological thing. By then the hunger of journalism had completely disappeared and I'd lost the intensity of only wanting a career. I felt there was more to life.

By the time I was 30, I was going through some terrible relationship traumas when one day I got a call from an old boyfriend, Andy, who was living and working in London.

'Come over here,' he said. 'Start your life afresh.' 'Oh yeah, sure,' I laughed. I hadn't seen him for five years. I had no idea what he looked like—he could have had no hair or a big stomach or God knows, something scary—but he'd always been a wonderful friend and very special.

Andy and I went out when we were both 24 and cub reporters at the ABC. He was the press gallery hack who loved political journalism and I was the journo who really just wanted to write. I took a job in the Northern Territory and although we tried the long-distance relationship, it was hard and neither of us wanted to move. I didn't think Canberra would be any good for my writing and he certainly didn't want to move to Alice Springs or Darwin. After a year, we decided there were other things more important to us at that stage of our lives. We were eager to taste the world, but we didn't split with bitterness and maintained a very strong friendship.

So when he rang, I teased, 'I'll just come over and check you out, mate', and left all the mess of my life behind in Australia. When I arrived, I found he was the same as he always was. It was lovely and I decided to stay with him in London.

Andy says he always knew I was the one, but it certainly took me by surprise and it really was wildly romantic. We lived in a little bedsit on Fleet Street for 18 months. He was doing night shifts at the Labour Party and I was doing them for the BBC World Service. I was also trying to write a novel in that tiny little room. And Andy's a television addict. So we thought if we could survive that one room, then maybe we could survive living together as husband and wife, and we were married in

Watsons Bay in Sydney on 30 December 1998.

I wanted children straight away but Andy was definite that he wanted a year of just us. So when January arrived the next year and we were flat-sitting in Paris, I was like, 'Wham bam! Here we go.' I'd put my legs above my head and hope everything fell into the right spot, but we didn't conceive there. We went to a friend's thirtieth birthday party back in London soon after, drank copious amounts of champagne, came home and conceived our first baby then.

I was really surprised as I thought it would take us a long time. I didn't have regular periods—sometimes my cycle would be five weeks, other times three months—and I wasn't a spring chicken. The midwives actually classified me as a mature mother on my first visit to London's Chelsea and Westminster Hospital—at the grand old age of 32.

I vomited the morning I bought the pregnancy test and I vomited all the way through to week 20. I vomited 17 times one day, a record. It used to come over me so quickly—I once went to the very chi-chi Notting Hill post office and had to run out of the queue to vomit in the gutter. But it was always happy vomiting. I felt a kind of strength in it. It made me feel the baby must have been lodged in there really securely for it to have such a reaction on me.

I was on a high the whole time I was pregnant. My God, my happy hormones—I adored them. I felt like I was on a drug and I'd never had anything like it before in my life. It was complete euphoria and I was in wonder that my body could do this.

And I felt really sexy. All my senses were heightened and so finely tuned. I was so womanly. I looked at myself in the mirror when I was heavily pregnant and naked and for the first time in my life thought, *I love my body. This is beautiful.* Normally, all I'd see were the faults, the fat thighs and tummy. I didn't want sex that much though—I was one of those women who just didn't feel like it—which was frustrating for Andy. But because we hadn't been married for long and we were both so joyous it was still like a blissful honeymoon anyway.

There were some physical discomforts. I have Rhesus-negative blood type, which meant I had to have injections throughout the pregnancy because the baby was likely to have a different blood type to me, and I was also low on iron. I took iron supplements and they were horrible—they made my stools black and revolting. But really, it was all by the by. It was a straightforward pregnancy, and I never saw a gyno or obstetrician. It was midwives all the way over here, which was great. They really know women.

I was working at the Beeb throughout the pregnancy and I finally had a doctor's exemption from those horrible 11-hour overnight shifts. And I was also solidly writing my third novel, *Lovesong*. The process was incredibly intensive. It went to 60 drafts and I was often up to three in the morning working. I finally finished it about a week before I was due as I didn't want to have the manuscript hanging around after the baby was born.

I was completely ignorant about birth. I didn't know anyone in London with a baby. All my friends were like me: professional women in their thirties, who'd come to London for careers and adventure, not to start families.

And I don't think I'd ever held a baby under three or four months old. I was always a bit scared of them and thought I'd drop them. So Andy and I went to every class we could find—in sheer terror. It was like, 'What on earth do we do?'

I soon decided I wanted a natural birth, if possible. I was keen on trying a water-birth as well—a good friend of mine in Australia had had one—but I was open to anything. I wasn't going to be a martyr in terms of pain. If it was going to be horrendous, then fine, I'd take the drugs. And if I needed to have an emergency Caesar, then fine as well. I was prepared for all contingencies. Whatever got me through.

I had a real craving for iron a week past the baby's due date in October 2000, so I ate a huge steak for dinner with Andy. Then, at three in the morning, I woke up to what felt like a little hand squeezing my tummy. I'd had Braxton Hicks contractions before, but this was very different.

I'd read every book in the world and had everything prepared—the birthing-ball, the stopwatch from the BBC. So I climbed out of bed, switched on CNN like the good journo I was, and sat on the ball with the stopwatch in my hand.

After only an hour, the contractions came on really quickly, so I rang the hospital, a busy, bustling government one. 'First-time mother?' asked the midwife. 'Oh, you'll be hours and hours.' 'I really think I should come in,' I said. 'No, no, no,' she replied. 'Just run a bath.'

So I ran a bath and I sat in it. But suddenly the contractions started to get really painful. 'Ring the hospital,' I yelled out to Andy. Again they told him it would be hours before I should go in. I knew what they were feeling. It was approaching six o'clock in the morning and their shift finished at eight. The last thing they wanted was another birthing woman to deal with.

It was amazing pain but I had absolutely no knowledge of what it was meant to be like. I kept thinking, *Okay, this is really painful but I've got another 24 hours of this.* There was no one there but Andy and me, and with the hospital saying I was going to be hours more, I assumed it was just meant to be this way.

I rang both Mum and Dad in Australia and Dad freaked out. 'What!' he said. 'Why aren't you in hospital? Get to hospital.' And all I could say was, 'But they're telling me I'm not allowed to.'

Eventually, I told Andy we were going to the hospital, no matter what, and on the third call they grudgingly said we could come in. So at seven o'clock, Andy got me in the car and we headed out into the middle of London morning traffic for Chelsea.

And all I wanted to do was rip off my clothes. It was a completely primal urge. I was scrambling at my cardigan and had to get everything off. I even tried to take off my wedding ring.

Andy started to get panicky and at a red light he put the child-locks on. Later he told me he thought I was going to just open up the door, clamber out and have the baby in the gutter. He also ran a red light.

We managed to swing around to pick up my girlfriend Bronnie at Bayswater and we were at the hospital in 20 minutes. As soon as I got into the room I took everything off and told the midwife I wanted a water-birth. She checked my cervix. 'There's no time to run a bath,' she said. 'You're fully dilated. Get on the bed and have this baby.' I had no idea I'd gone that far. It was all so quick.

We'd brought the birthing-ball, had all the cassettes and the candles, but I just climbed onto the bed and instinctively squatted, with my hands over the bedhead. It was a natural position for me. 'Yep,' said the midwife. 'Go for it.'

Andy, God love him, was saying, 'Oh my God, what do I do?', whereas Bronnie, who'd never been through anything like this before either, just automatically, as a woman I guess, started giving me water and rubbing the small of my back.

This animal thing kicked in and I surrendered to my body entirely. I let nature take over and allowed my body to do it all without rationalising or fighting it. It was telling me, 'Yes, it's painful, but yes, I can handle this and it feels right.' And after all these years, I was listening to my body. I felt in control even though I had never done this before. I actually felt like a she-wolf who'd gone off to a lair in the hills.

I held Andy's hand on the side of the bed and was sucking away on the gas and biting down on the plastic nozzle really hard. But I don't think I felt any great pain relief. It certainly didn't feel like when you go to the dentist and you're all happy and out of it.

My tummy felt like a huge sponge, squeezing downwards in a spiral, but it wasn't until the baby entered the birth canal and I started pushing that I felt I was literally on a rack being torn apart. *Nikki*, I thought, completely rationally, *you are never, ever doing this again*. It was like a little mental note to myself.

My midwife, Eve, was amazing. I may have been listening to my body but when it came to the end of the pushing, I was listening to her like a good little schoolgirl. The darling was trying to stop me from tearing and I was desperate for her to stop me tearing too.

And then, at 8.08 a.m., Lachlan came out, screaming and bright pink, and Eve put him straight to my breast. Both of us were completely messy and shitty and bloody, and as he started suckling, I looked down and thought, *It's like a little alien there. How does he instantly know to do this?* And at that moment, I'd never felt more empowered, more strong, more womanly and female. It was the most exhilarating and joyous feeling.

It was such a lovely atmosphere in there with just the five of us—the baby, Andy, Bronnie, Eve and me. Eve asked Andy if he wanted to cut the umbilical cord but he didn't want to go near it. 'Come on you,' she said, and he reluctantly did it. Unfortunately I tore and Eve said, 'I'll stitch you up nice and tight.' I thought *Oh my God, do I really want that?* I actually found the constipation and the pain of the stitches much more difficult to deal with afterwards than the pain of the birth. There was a wonderful end-result after labour, but the stitches were just annoying.

I looked over at Andy sitting beside me just holding and holding Lachie, who was all swaddled up. It was like the supreme moment of his life. He was entirely focused on this little tiny creature and it was as if I had disappeared completely from his world.

Once our midwife left—she'd stayed past the end of her shift to see Lachlan born—the hospital told us they wanted us out in six hours. Andy and I were horrified, but that's the way it is in England. It had been a very quick, straightforward labour and birth with minimal tearing, so they wanted us out. We were a statistic and they needed the bed.

I was really scared and we begged them to let us stay. 'I don't know how to hold him or bathe him,' I said. Thankfully, they gave us that one night and I shared a room with seven other women. I was so tired and I woke up in the middle of the night to Lachie screaming. He'd done a poo and vomited up a lot of mucus so it was all happening from both ends and I looked at him and just thought, *Where do I begin*? Thank God the night nurse was there to help.

We went home the next morning and we really had no idea what we were doing. A community nurse came out on day three and day six and weighed and checked Lachlan and, I don't know why, but I didn't feel comfortable enough to ask all those basic questions about feeding and crying. And I had no friends or family over here to show me what to do.

Before I left the hospital, one of the midwives had said to me, 'Nikki, you are amongst the most disadvantaged of mothers.' And I asked her why. 'You're a middle-class professional ex-pat,' she said. 'Women like you have no one around to help. You would have been so much better off if you were a single mother on a council estate in London because you'd have had a huge amount of support.'

I rang up my mum in Australia when Lachie was about five or six days old. 'Mum, he's crying all the time and I don't know what to do,' I said. 'Well, have you burped him?' she asked. 'What?' I didn't know what she was talking about. 'Just pat his back, darling, to kind of wind him after he's had some milk.' And I said, 'Ooohhh.'

I really felt out of control just after Lachlan was born, and that was a first for me. In a way, my whole adult life had been about control. My parents divorced when I was young and my mother, who raised me, once told me, 'Never rely on a man, Nikki. You must always be able to make your own way in the world.' I controlled my career, I had my own place, mortgage and car from a very young age, and it wasn't until I had Lachie, at 33, that suddenly it was like, 'Oh, whoa. I have to relinquish all this control.'

I also lost a lot of confidence. I was supposed to go back to work after three months and I thought, *I can't walk into that newsroom and sit at that terminal and produce a program. I can't do that.* And I'd lost confidence in my writing. *Lovesong* had been so intense—I used to write 16 hours a day sometimes—and I knew there was no way I could work like that with a little baby. I just didn't have the energy, stamina or brainpower.

I spoke to my sister-in-law and a good girlfriend in Australia a lot during those first few weeks. 'I don't know how to do this,' I'd tell them. And they both told me about the Sydney family care centre, Tresillian. I rang them all the way from London and said, 'I need a bit of guidance here.'

They booked me in for a live-in week in January, so we flew home a couple of months after Lachlan was born to see the family for Christmas—and for Tresillian.

And it was fantastic. It was like I needed blunt, matter-of-fact Aussie women around me to tell me what to do. They helped give me some control over the situation and also let me sleep because I was completely exhausted. I emerged from there confident as a mum and that compensated for everything else. *I can do this now*, I thought.

We jumped on a plane and when I got back to London I was energised and champing at the bit to start a new book. And because I was high on hormones and having no sex, I felt like writing a book about sex in marriage. There was an intense physicality to pregnancy and being a new mother and I wanted to channel that heightened awareness. So that was the atmosphere that brewed *The Bride Stripped Bare*.

But it was a completely different experience for me. I would run up to my little desk by our bed and snatch an hour or two while Lachlan slept. I'd write from nine o'clock at night, but I couldn't work very intensely because I was so tired. I'd get to about eleven or twelve and my brain would just go.

I had no time to indulge or dwell, so it was a very different way of writing and that's why the book was written in very short chapters—the first was only four lines long—and is very linear. I wasn't getting bogged down in complexity.

And no one except Andy and a few close friends knew I was writing. My agent, my parents and my publisher all had no idea. They all assumed I'd stepped into babyland and would be gone for a couple of years. And that was liberating. I had this void ahead of me that gave me an exhilarating, reckless freedom to do whatever I wanted. I was in a trance-like little bubble of isolation and babies and I thought I could have some fun, and if it didn't work I could shelve it and put it in a bottom drawer somewhere.

I was also in some strange ego-less existence and didn't feel I needed to have my name attached to it.

It was a lovely, experimental, rich time of my life. And I must admit the only time I felt completely in control during the madness of a new baby was when I was sitting at my writing desk. Those moments never lasted long, but they were enough. They calmed me and strengthened me to be able to go back to the chaos of my wonderful, messy world with little Lachie and Andy. I guess they were moments of pure selfishness.

I really didn't come down for ages after having Lachie. Both Andy and I found the whole process wondrous and wonderful and it gave me incredible confidence as a woman. It also made me addicted to having more kids.

In September 2001, I went to Sydney for the Australian launch of *Lovesong*. I was catching up with an old friend just before I was due to fly back to London when suddenly I felt really tired. *I know this exhaustion*, I thought. *I know what it is.* I bought a pregnancy testing kit at Kingsford Smith airport, did the test in the loo and it came up positive.

It was two o'clock in the morning in London and I rang Andy and told him. We were both absolutely delighted, but it certainly took me by surprise. Lachie was only nine months old and I was still breastfeeding. I didn't like the idea of those long flights so early in the pregnancy. I probably would have cancelled the *Lovesong* book tour had I known I was pregnant.

The second pregnancy was a lot more exhausting than the first. I had the same kind of euphoria but I wasn't looking after myself as well as I did that first time and I had a toddler to run after. I was also desperately trying to finish *Bride* before the baby was born, but it just wasn't ready.

My midwife thought I might not make it to the hospital this time because of Lachie's quick birth, so towards the end of the pregnancy she schooled me on how to have a home birth. She said I'd need to heat up some towels because newborns started to lose body heat really quickly and she also told me not to touch the umbilical cord; the ambulance crew would deal with that.

So when contractions violently woke me up at one o'clock in the morning on 29 May 2002, I was prepared. I got out all the towels and started putting them over the heaters, but ten minutes or so down the track I stopped. *What am I doing?* I thought. *I can't do this. I can't go through this alone at home with just Andy and Lachie.*

We didn't have any family to leave Lachie with, so Andy grabbed him and bundled us into the car. When we arrived at the hospital the staff was really cross we'd brought our 18 month old, but we had no choice.

I was fully dilated again and while Andy parked the car and organised Lachie, my body just clicked into motion. This time I actually recognised what it was doing ahead of the midwives and by the time Andy arrived, Oliver was plopping onto the bed. We made it to the hospital with just 17 minutes to spare and it was only an hour and ten minutes from first contraction to birth. Lachlan slept through the whole thing in his pram in a spare birthing suite next door.

I tore again and told the midwife I didn't want stitches. It had been so painful with Lachlan and I thought leaving it to heal naturally would be better. But that was a big mistake. It took longer to heal and it was awful.

Although both births were natural, I must admit there is the journalist and writer in me who wouldn't mind having a Caesarean. I'd love to try the alternative, just to experience it and compare. And I would love to have another baby. There's actually something in me that would love five, but I'm gettin' on. And if I did have another one it would probably be like, don't even bother getting in the car.

I'd always been scared that having children would impede me as a writer. But as a mother, I'm at the coalface of living and that can be a really good place to be. Becoming a mother has taught me so much about human nature and has been a very rich experience for me as a writer. But really, writing has now been pushed to the periphery of my life. It's my babies that fill up my world.

Postscript

Nikki Gemmell never returned to the BBC after having Lachlan in 2000. She extended her maternity leave to six months, then to a year, before finally resigning after a 'career break' when he was 18 months old.

In October 2002, four months after giving birth to Oliver, Nikki's erotic postnatal writing project, *The Bride Stripped Bare*, became the focus of a bidding war at the Frankfurt Book Fair. It went on to become the top-selling adult novel in Australia for 2003 and an international bestseller.

The novel also immersed Nikki, who wrote the book anonymously, in controversy after she was exposed as its author. She says she decided to remove her name from novel to protect the people closest to her. 'It was that broody mother hen thing,' she adds. 'I didn't want anything to crash into the serenity of our tiny little unit.'

But unfortunately, it did. 'Some of the mothers at Lachie's nursery still give me a look like "We know what you're like",' says Nikki. 'But I've reached the stage of my life where I won't be held hostage to what other people think of me.'

While she admits it's hard to imagine her sons reading her intensely personal and often explicit work, she says she is 'so deep into their world at the moment, it's like, whatever. I'm sure it will be fine'.

Nikki is now working on another novel entitled *The Book of Pleasure*, plus a sequel to *Bride*, and has a strong yearning to return to Australia. 'I've done what I've needed to do career-wise,' says the author, who was born in Wollongong, New South Wales. 'I want to be amongst my family and friends and the land.' However, her husband Andrew Sholl, a public relations consultant, is still keen on the family living in London.

In the meantime, she is accustoming her boys, the older of whom has an English accent, to all things Australian through DVDs of the 1970s classic *Skippy*. The only downside is that this makes Nikki even more homesick than she already is.

My great unknown adventure

SALLY MACHIN

My father was diagnosed with cancer in the middle of 2000 and I realised at the time that I needed to simplify my life in order to cope with his dying. I stopped smoking and going out drinking every night and really focused on my diet. I also stopped putting too much emotional energy into my work as a corporate lawyer.

My father died in the middle of the Sydney 2000 Olympics, and by default Gary and I found ourselves in the right place to have a baby. I'd changed my lifestyle and after working for a few years in London I was back in Sydney where I wanted to be. Gary and I had bought a family home in a family neighbourhood, my brother had recently had a child and my father's death made me much more family minded.

I wasn't somebody who ever dreamt about weddings and children and white picket fences, but we were very happy when we found out I was pregnant in early 2001. Must have been that festive Christmas party season.

I'd cut out a lot of my old vices so didn't really need to give anything up but I was still working pretty solidly. And I decided early on in the pregnancy that the pregnancy was not going to affect me or my work: I'd just carry on as normal, working 60-hour weeks and travelling overnight on long-haul flights every three weeks or so for my regional role. The one kind of food I couldn't stand early in the pregnancy was curry and when I was 12 weeks pregnant, I was sent to India. I hadn't told anyone yet and I just thought, *I can't be sick, I can't say anything to anyone, I can't stop work for two seconds*, and ate the plainest meals I could find.

The people at my company were actually fine when I eventually told them. I was 33, had been married for three or four years and it was very much expected. But I wasn't about to make any concessions. I thought people would judge me if I left work at 6 p.m. and felt that the company had all these expectations, but really, I think I made them up in my head. I didn't have the confidence to realise that people actually wanted me for my experience, expertise and efficiency rather than the hours I put in or the fact I was superwoman.

I stopped flying at seven months but only because I was told to. The airlines and travel insurance wouldn't cover me after that, but there were stories going around about some woman who'd flown when she was eight months pregnant wearing an overcoat to hide her stomach. It was like a badge of honour and part of the 'I'm tougher than anyone else' mentality and I was very much caught up in that.

Besides a bit of bleeding at 20 weeks, I had an absolute

breeze of a pregnancy and I really had no birth plan of any description; I just hadn't given it any thought. I was incredibly disorganised and by the time I got around to booking antenatal classes it was too late to get into one other than six weeks before my due date. I did the minimal amount of preparation I possibly could.

My baby was breech, so I did briefly talk to my obstetrician about what the options would be if the baby didn't move. 'Do you want to go into a program to try and turn the baby to give birth naturally?' she asked. I knew the success rate of these programs was low and I'd probably have to skip more work if I went into one. I already had to go to obstetrician appointments every few weeks, so I thought I'd probably opt for a Caesarean. *I couldn't possibly take more time off work*, I thought. But no decisions were made—we were just going to wait and see if the baby turned by itself.

Gary was studying sports science and his sister was getting married in England around the baby's due date. His uni holidays were coming up, so I said, 'Why don't you go back to England and try to see everybody anyway?' He thought it was a good idea, so we used my frequent flyer points and I sent him on his way in early July when I was 33 weeks pregnant.

A week later, we moved down a floor at work. I'd been shifting boxes—as you do at 34 weeks—and when I had a sore back the next day I put it down to the lifting. But when I went to the bathroom at around 10 o'clock that morning I saw some bleeding, and I'd read enough to know that back pain *and* bleeding was not a great combination.

My obstetrician was away, so I rang her partner. 'I think I probably need to see someone,' I said, and the receptionist booked me in for five o'clock that afternoon.

The back pain continued throughout the day. My obstetrician had warned me when I'd had that earlier bleed that I might need bed rest. I thought, at worst, I might need to be in hospital for a day or two, so my assistant and I started making preparations just in case. She got a set of spare keys cut for home and we started putting little notes on files.

I stayed at work the entire day even though my backache was getting worse and then I went to my afternoon appointment in Newtown. 'I'm having a little bit of back pain,' I told the obstetrician. 'Do you think I could take a Panadol?' For me to ask for Panadol was probably like someone else asking for pethidine, and my usual obstetrician would have known straight away that something was wrong. But I'd never been to this doctor before and he obviously got the wrong impression of the degree of pain I was in.

He gave me an internal examination, told me my cervix was intact and that the bleed could have been a number of things. He said I was having Braxton Hicks contractions but seemed to think everything was fine and advised me to go home and rest. *Okay*, I thought. *I've got a while to go yet.*

Usually I'd take a bus back home from the obstetrician's, but that day I decided to take a cab. It was early evening and when I got home I felt lousy and wanted to go to bed, but Gary was due to call from England and there was also a 10 o'clock conference call I needed to stay up for. My back was killing me but I'd really pushed a manager into holding this call so I knew I had to do it.

Gary didn't phone and by the time 10 o'clock came around and I made the work call in my study, I was racked with excruciating pain. I still didn't know what it was but I'd read somewhere that rocking could help. So there I was rocking back and forth on all fours while trying to contribute in a meaningful way to the call with colleagues in New York, London and Geneva. I was very short of temper.

Finally, 11 o'clock came. *Right*, I thought. *An hour's up. I'll be able to go.* But someone said the obligatory, 'Does anybody have anything else to talk about?' and my American colleague decided to go into this verbose discussion about a takeover he was working on. I absolutely adored him but all I wanted to say was, 'Shut the fuck up.' I remained silent except for the odd comment and I rocked there for another half hour with him droning on about a very important issue—just one I wasn't in the mood to listen to.

It was finally over by 11.30 p.m. I was so tired that all I wanted to do was go to bed, but when I climbed in and lay there, I couldn't sleep. *I'm sure I've seen something on television about contractions*, I thought. *It's not really good if they're regular, particularly if these are contractions.* My sister-in-law had given me the only book I had—*Baby Love*—so I went and got that and read it, but I still didn't think they were contractions.

The pain was all around my back and I was convinced contractions needed to be in the front. I started timing the pain anyway and it was four minutes apart. *Right*, I thought.

Who should I phone? My husband wasn't there, my best friend, who was supposed to be my birth partner, was in Melbourne and my mother had just flown home to Tasmania. *I can't possibly phone my obstetrician—it's the middle of the night*, I thought, so I looked for the hospital's number and phoned the midwife in the delivery suite. 'I think you'd better come in,' she said.

I'd always had this vision of my husband racing me to the hospital, but he wasn't there and I had to think really hard about how I was going to get there. Eventually, I rang a cab. 'I need to go to the Mater Hospital,' I said politely. 'Are you ready now?' said the telephonist. 'Oh yes,' I replied, and she told me that she'd send the next available cab. 'Do you think you might be able to put a bit of priority against it?' I asked. Obviously someone knew what the Mater was and what my call at that time of the night might mean, because a very nice cab driver turned up a couple of minutes later.

I switched off all the lights, locked the house and walked outside in my tracksuit and ugg boots—back when they were strictly something you didn't wear out of the house—with a bag I'd thrown together earlier in the day. 'Going to work, are you?' said the cabbie. *In my ugg boots?* I thought. 'No,' I said. 'I actually think I'm in labour.'

A woman in labour is probably a taxi driver's nightmare, or dream, and I could see the excitement on his face. 'Do you want me to drive fast or do you want me to drive carefully?' he asked. 'Carefully would be good,' I replied. But really, it wouldn't have mattered what I'd said, because he drove at the rate of knots through a midnight blanket of fog with me lying in the back trying to hold a conversation. He was a taxi driver, so of course he was talking, but silly me was trying to talk back.

I arrived at the hospital at about 12.30 a.m. After the midwife admitted me, she immediately hooked me up to everything and it became bleatingly obvious I was having contractions. She was concerned about the bleeding and had a sense that this was going to be a difficult birth, so she called my stand-in obstetrician.

The pain was worse than anything I'd ever experienced and all I wanted was drugs, but because they didn't know what was going on they wouldn't let me have anything: no gas, no Panadol, nothing. I hadn't done any research so I didn't really know the options that well, but I knew I needed those drugs.

'We've rung the doctor,' the midwife kept saying. 'He's coming in.' 'Is he bringing his drugs?' was all I could say. I was like a petulant child after a while. I wouldn't speak to her unless she was offering drugs and nobody was allowed to see me unless they had them. But she was amazing. She was obviously warding off this impending tantrum that would come as soon as somebody actually told me I wasn't allowed any drugs. She would have made a great nanny.

I used to sing a song from *The Sound of Music* to try and calm down an asthmatic girlfriend during an attack, so I quickly found myself sitting on that bed alone, singing, 'Raindrops on roses and whiskers on kittens . . .'

My doctor soon arrived and although he was trying very hard to make it appear that I had choices, it was obvious I needed to have an emergency Caesarean. 'We don't really know what's causing this unspecified bleeding,' he kept saying. 'It could be a number of things.' He was being very evasive and after a while I asked him bluntly, 'Is the baby in danger?'

'Yes.'

'What's the best way of getting the baby out of danger? Would we have time to deliver naturally?'

'Well, no.'

'So we have to do a Caesarean?'

'Yes.'

'Well, do one,' I said. I couldn't really understand why we were even talking about it.

I had to make these decisions by myself but it was easy for me to do. I didn't have any baggage about birth plans or preconceived ideas, and this obstetrician had grey hair and was 50. He was experienced—I'd earlier sat in his waiting room and a pregnant 18-year-old girl came in who he'd delivered 18 years ago—so I just let him get on with it and he started ringing the various crews to get them out of bed and into the hospital.

At that stage, no one close to me knew where I was or what was happening. I'd spoken to my sister-in-law earlier in the day—she had her suspicions I was having contractions, even though I didn't—and she told me to ring any time of the day or night. It was fortunate she did because otherwise I would have never thought to call.

I rang and spoke to my brother, Scott. 'Can you please come over?' I asked between contractions. 'I'm here by myself and they're about to deliver my baby by emergency Caesarean.'

He was very excited. They'd recently had a baby and he'd missed out on the emergency dash across to the hospital—it was quite full at the time and the staff had told them not to rush in. Now it was three o'clock in the morning, his sister was about to have an emergency Caesar by herself, and he was there in what seemed like five minutes.

They moved me into the operating theatre and by that stage, I couldn't have given a stuff. I was signing paperwork and asking everyone who came near me, 'Have you got the drugs? Are you the anaesthetist?' I was totally focused on those drugs and I think I was completely gone by then.

The anaesthetist eventually arrived and gave me a quick-working local anaesthetic because it was too late for an epidural. I thought he was the most wonderful man in the world and I wanted to have his children by then! Once it was done I had this incredible feeling of relief. 'Oh, thank God,' I said.

Scott soon had his doctor's kit and mask on and was running around thinking he was quite the baby expert. He stood right beside me—brothers are strictly up the hand-holding end—and it all happened really quickly. It was 4.15 a.m. and the next thing I knew they'd pulled out Jessica. I didn't get to hold her—I hardly even saw her. The nurse just walked past me, held up the baby and headed straight for neonatal intensive care.

The baby weighed five pounds five ounces and went straight into an oxygen tent but she was fine. Scott started taking photos and went with her and suddenly half the people in the room had disappeared. The doctor and his assistant were the only people there and they were sewing me up and chatting away between themselves.

The pain had gone and I knew the baby was safe and all of a sudden it hit me and the loneliness really kicked in.

I had an overwhelming sense of 'this is not how it's meant to be', and I began to cry. *This is all wrong,* I thought, as the tears fell down my face. *Where's my husband? Where's my mother? Where is everybody?* No one was there for me and I lay on my own with these two men talking about golf.

The doctors didn't say anything—I'm sure they'd seen it all before—and by the time I got back to the ward it was practically morning and I still felt like I had no idea what was going on. The baby was in neonatal intensive care up the hallway—they later wheeled me in to see her—Scott was off ringing my mum and trying to track Gary down, and I was soon throwing up over the side of the bed because of the pethidine. I didn't have an epidural so they couldn't drip-feed the drug and they'd given it to me as an injection in the leg. It was like a big hit and I really was in cuckoo-land.

My mum was busy trying to organise a flight from Tasmania and Gary's parents eventually tracked him down, surfing in Cornwall. He called at nine o'clock that morning. I was completely exhausted but by then he was having a ball in the pub, celebrating and smoking cigars.

And then I rang work. My assistant Sarah was mortified I'd gone into labour at work—it was her absolute fear I would give birth there—but she was even more horrified when I asked her to bring in my laptop and refused, point-blank, despite my pleadings.

It had happened so fast. I didn't really know this baby—I'd seen her for about two seconds—and my thoughts immediately turned to work. I felt like I should be in the office. I thought I was completely irreplaceable and Sarah came in that afternoon and I gave her instructions about where to delegate my work and when I'd be available—and she also brought in that computer.

It was all so unexpected that it really caused a stir at work. I'd walked out the door one afternoon and the next morning I'd had a baby. There were lots of phone calls, flowers and people dropping in. It really was a natural continuation with the way I had been living my life, but I'd just had major surgery and it soon became out of control. I was trying to get up out of bed but couldn't and I didn't have anyone to control the situation. Mum arrived later that afternoon and even though she was a great support, she didn't really know my friends, who wanted to speak to me and weren't going to be satisfied with just talking to 'the mother'.

I hadn't done any of the antenatal classes—my first one was booked for the day after Jessica was born—so I didn't realise I was meant to start breastfeeding straight away. The midwives had sort of forgotten about me and I was on the phone and doing what I was doing but after a while it occurred to somebody that the baby needed food and I needed to be milked. So all of a sudden people came in and I sat there with midwives trying to squeeze colostrum out of my breasts and into little tubes.

Gary finally arrived back on the Sunday and he was there for day four when the baby blues arrived and Jessica became jaundiced. I was so glad he was there—he's got a great sense of humour and laughed at everything, even as Jessica lay in the light-box with her 'sunglasses' on. It was very hard to get too deeply into emotional distress when I had somebody who made everything quite amusing.

I was glad Gary wasn't there for the birth though. He's very scientific and he would have wanted to have known the answers. But the doctors didn't have any. They couldn't give enough information to make an informed, rational decision, and I think he would have gone off because nobody could tell him what was going on. My obstetrician later told me that obstetrics was an art not a science—and I was in so much pain I didn't really care what decisions were made.

Jessica was fed through a tube for that first week and I didn't get to take her home with me when I left after six days. I travelled twice a day back to the hospital to feed her and be with her but it really took me a couple of weeks to recover from the Caesarean.

She was in hospital for 17 days and I took six weeks off before I started working one day a week. I took four and a half months off in all and then Gary, who was on a uni break, looked after Jessica for three months. We were a single-income family and we had a large mortgage to pay, so I didn't have any choice about when to go back to work. But I probably would have gone anyway. There's really not much to do with first babies once you're over that three-month hurdle. It's actually hard to fill your day. You really need maternity leave with toddlers—they can fill your day any time.

I was happy to go back to work, but it took a while for me to gain the confidence to realise I didn't have to be there late at night to get my job done. The company went through a cost-cutting process and travel was restricted, and luckily I had a manager who was very Zen. He helped change my approach and made me realise that if I had confidence in my team and could let go a bit, the world wouldn't fall apart. I did that and found it worked.

I fell pregnant with my second child a few months after Jessica's first birthday and work was very accepting again. Then, at my 18-week scan, the doctors found a tear in my cervix, which could have caused an infection and induced labour. After weekly monitoring for a month it became obvious it wasn't going to improve, so my obstetrician told me I would either need bed rest for the rest of the pregnancy in the hope the baby would reach its survival date, or he could put a stitch in my cervix. The stitch was risky—it was a foreign object and could itself trigger labour—but I had one put in at 23 weeks.

I had to have an epidural to have it done and it was a straightforward process. I was in hospital for four days but there was really no recovery and afterwards I sat in the hospital feeling well but bored out of my brain and immediately started negotiating my release. But it was obvious this specialist was used to dealing with women like me. He'd bring six students with him every time he had to tell me something, especially if it involved me not going anywhere.

There was still a high risk I could go into early labour. The odds were a straight 50-50 and they were horrible. I was working full time and couldn't take any time off work—I needed to save four weeks annual leave to string out the length of time I could have with the baby—and I had full-on nerves until 28 weeks, which was the first viable date. I counted down those weeks and each week I'd read about what a premature baby born at that stage in the pregnancy would end up like. So although the baby stayed there, it was a stressful pregnancy, and probably as a result I got back pain for the remainder of it.

My doctor told me I could possibly try for a natural birth but there were always going to be potential complications from the scarring of the previous birth, and I probably would've ended up having a Caesarean anyway. They also had to take the stitch out at 38 weeks. I thought it would have been weird going in for that procedure and then going home to wait for labour, and in the back of my mind I knew I wanted to work as long as I could to spend more time with the baby.

The stitch worked and my doctor booked me in for the Caesarean on 14 August 2003. I gave myself one day off work and had a good night's sleep before the operation. I was very relaxed the next morning. The bag was packed, the nanny was there to look after Jessica and Gary drove me to the hospital.

And when I arrived, I knew how things worked. I was familiar with the operating theatre, recognised all the forms and knew what drugs I wanted. It was all very easy this time, and I wasn't in any pain when they put the epidural in.

The operation was very civilised and it seemed to take a lot longer than last time. I suppose they hacked in there that first time to get Jessica out as quickly as possible whereas this time it was a gentle sort of carving, layer by layer.

Gary stayed with me, and he was fascinated. The doctor let him down the business end and explained everything as he did it. It was so good having him there. My recollection of Jessica's birth was quite hazy. Without someone there to tell me what had happened, it kind of felt like 'Did that really happen?' This time, Gary could tell me it did and (apart from the photos he took of me up in stirrups) it felt more like it was meant to have been.

My recovery was much quicker with Ruby and the baby got to room in with me, which was so different. I was mobile and the pethidine this time was drip-fed and much more bearable. After a couple of days I told the midwives I wanted to go straight on to Panadol, as last time Panadeine Forte had made me constipated and it was horrible. This time I knew what I wanted and the births were like two completely different operations. The second just wasn't as tough as that first time.

I look back on Jessica's birth and I really think I was stark raving mad. I was bonkers and it just makes me laugh. Everything about it was stupid: not knowing I was in labour, not telling the cab driver to haul his arse over to my place straight away, not calling my obstetrician at midnight, having that conference call. But I have no regrets—it's not in my nature—and I don't feel like one of life's great experiences has passed me by.

Women have so many expectations when they're pregnant and everything is so focused on them. There is so much pressure about the experience your child is going to have and how you'll scar them for life if you don't do it the right way. But you can scar your children in lots of other ways that no one seems interested in telling you about. There's no right way and wrong way of doing this. And once you've got those babies, they're the most precious things in the world and it doesn't matter how they got here.

I think of birth as one of the few great adventures left in life. What else do you have absolutely no ability to control? You can try and help and plan and all that stuff's good, but when it comes down to it, you can't control it. You just have to kick back and say, 'My great unknown adventure.'

Postscript

Shortly after returning to work from three-and-a-half months' maternity leave with her second baby, Ruby, Sally Machin discovered she was pregnant with her third child. 'The first time I did my six-week postnatal check-up, I thought it was such a waste of time,' she says. 'So I skipped this one. The point I missed was that at that check-up the doctor puts you back on contraception.'

While she and Gary, who now works in sports science, were very happy with their surprise, Sally noticed a different response from her colleagues. Her third child was expected to be 13 months older than her second and this, it seems, was not quite what they thought would happen. 'It's been very odd,' Sally says. 'There's been a lot of disapproval with people saying things like, "I suppose I should congratulate you."'

And people seem to think she is now a 'real' mother. 'A mother of one or two fits into the image of a working mother but once you're up to three, four or five it's like, "You must really like kids, you're not just having them because you're meant to."'

To cope with her hectic life, Sally has 'teams of other people', including a live-in nanny and cleaners, to help and says she has learnt to 'disengage from things that are not important' such as a tidy home and office politics. 'I think you either get more stressed or more laid back,' she says. 'I've relinquished a lot of control and worked out which battles to fight.'

And it is lucky she has: Sally went into early labour with her third child and on 31 July 2004, William Fynn Osborne was delivered by emergency Caesarean, seven weeks early. William joined his elder sisters at home after 24 days in hospital. 'The problem this time was identical to that with my first child and completely different from the problems with my second,' says Sally. 'My obstetrician said he could write a book about me and was hoping I'd have more children.' But that, adds Sally, is unlikely at this stage.

Into his arms

JENNY ANN COOK

My parents were living in North Ryde and already had three children, so Mum had plenty of experience with birth. When she woke up in the middle of the night at the end of her fourth pregnancy and said, 'We've got to go to the hospital now,' she wasn't sure the ambulance would come in time. It did, but on the way to Darlinghurst's St Margaret's Hospital my dad, who's a doctor, tapped on the window to make the driver stop. I came out in a real rush and my father caught me. Mum and Dad knew there were a lot of cars around but it wasn't until the ambulance moved on again that they realised where they'd stopped. I was born on the Sydney Harbour Bridge.

I didn't find out until I was about 11. We were sitting out in the sun eating iceblocks with our best family friends and everyone was telling stories about when they were born. When Dad said, 'Well, Jenny was born on the Harbour Bridge,' we all stopped talking and looked at him. We were like, 'What?' Mum said she didn't want to tell me earlier because she thought I'd be embarrassed, but by that age I was very iconic and proud to be Australian so to be born on an icon was quite amazing. And as I grew older, I thought it was lovely to have been born high above water. For a long time my notion of birth was all tied up with iceblocks out the back.

In my teens, I was an innocent in many ways. I studied economics at uni at the suggestion of others and joined the public service when I left. My family was thrilled and the first few years were terrific. I loved my job and colleagues and saw myself as a long-term worker for the public good. But I started to flounder when the depression I had felt occasionally as a youngster crept back in. Work became more political with promotion and I felt the public was being misled. I became incredibly disillusioned and anxious and one day I walked out and never went back.

I was quite a wreck after that—I couldn't answer the phone for months and lost friends rather than explain what had happened. I was sad that I was giving up the world that a lot of people had thought was right for me and I also felt ashamed to be unemployed.

Later I found part-time work and the easy-come, easy-go nature of that suited me well. I was happy to sleep in the morning and work at night and spent lots of time in the pub and the library.

One night in 1994 I was visiting a musician friend when this guy walked in wearing white overalls and a baseball cap with his long hair tucked in, giving him this crazy fringe. I'd heard about this new flatmate, Ian, but didn't know he had been to a fancy dress party. He was a bit drunk and stumbled around and grabbed a guitar and started singing some noisy songs he'd composed. He made a good impression and soon started coming over to my house every day.

Ian was gorgeous but some of my friends didn't like him. He was younger—I was 26, he was 20—and he was supposedly a westie. He'd wear his Metallica T-shirt all the time and I liked that he was musical, a vegetarian and had long hair—his mother told me later that he hadn't let her cut it since he was 12.

We had great fun together. 'How long is this going to go on?' I'd say. 'Forever, Jenny,' he'd say, and I'd laugh at that. But soon we were driving around the countryside in his old Holden panel van and a few months later we were on a flight to Kathmandu.

By early 1997, Ian and I were back in Australia, living in Stuart Park on the neck of the Darwin Peninsula. There were lots of young families in Darwin. It was a hot, tropical climate and there was easy employment. As suburbia goes, it was wild suburbia: the house was surrounded by louvres and it sat on a giant block of land filled with mango trees. We were having a lovely time and I started pestering Ian for a baby. I was incredibly hormonal. I'd be desperate around ovulation time and would be in tears when my period came. Ian tried to reason with me: 'I'm too young, can't you wait?' But I persisted and one day Ian, who was by then 23, said, 'Yeah, all right.'

The night I conceived our baby was the best night of my life and I knew straight away. It was as warm as could be and I went out into the big backyard and sat under the full moon and thanked the gods and the angels and prayed, especially to Mary, Our Lady of the Rosary. Ian didn't believe I was pregnant, but I wasn't mistaken. Soon my breasts were big, my period was overdue and I was thrilled. *Right, that's it*, I thought and I never had a test.

Not long into the pregnancy, I decided to cash in my superannuation from the public service and take Ian to South-east Asia. We went to Thailand, travelled down through Malaysia and got the boat across to Indonesia. We lived quite simply. I had two sarongs, two cotton shirts and a pair of sandals, and Ian's small bag was bursting with books. Hotel rooms were small and cheap and lunch and dinner were rice, greens and tofu. I did yoga in the space by the bed and most days we would walk for miles. I felt fit and healthy.

We returned to Australia in October with a six-month baby bump and decided to go bush. We bought a mosquito net and a $1000 van and drove to the Cox Peninsula where a friend of ours, Mick, lived in a stone house he'd built on Aboriginal land with the permission of the local community. Mick was a former miner, construction worker and Builders Labourers Federation organiser and was full of stories and loved to entertain. We camped about half a kilometre away from him and slept on the sandy flat of this huge escarpment. It was rugged land and at night I'd usually cook us all rice and lentils with lots of spice and sweet potatoes. Town was a two-hour drive away or a 30-minute ferry ride and every fortnight I'd go in for a fresh fruit fix.

It was easy living and it was beautiful. I did yoga every day, and in the evenings hundreds of white cockatoos would slowly fly by, calling to each other. There would always be stragglers. Kookaburras were often laughing and the blue on their wings made them look like the sky.

But the sandflies were amazing. In shady hours I'd walk around and have this little cloud on my feet. Once I bent down and it was as if someone had put a velvet pillow on my face as the sandflies settled on my skin. They had a very itchy bite so I soon bought some long-sleeved men's cotton shirts from an op-shop and although it was hot, I'd wear them with trakky daks and be covered from my ankles to my wrists.

I didn't think I needed to see any doctors throughout the pregnancy. I felt I'd had a fair bit of exposure to their world when I was growing up. I had quite a few doctors in my immediate and extended family and I was no longer in awe of the medical profession or what it could do for me. I always felt that if I was healthy, which I was, and felt all right, which I did, then what benefit would medical interference be?

I'd borrowed some books from the Darwin library, which were all written by male doctors, and they were horrific. They talked about ways to hold forceps and said things like, 'Don't worry if the child has clamp marks on its head.' That confirmed my decision that I wasn't going to let anybody near my belly. And Ian was really firm about it. 'Put those stupid books away,' he'd say. 'I'm not going to let them have a go at you.' I'd also met a woman who'd given birth on a beach in Thailand. Her daughter was now a big, healthy teenager and that helped me realise that birth wasn't something to fear.

I was very superstitious throughout the pregnancy. I hadn't wanted people knowing, including my family back in Sydney. I didn't want anyone trying to take the power by saying, 'For my sake, please go to the doctor.' I felt that this was Ian's and my baby and we wanted it to come out healthy and strong. And that's what I prayed for. I didn't ask for a girl or a smartie. I didn't ask for anything but healthy and strong.

We drove down to Batchelor, about two hours away on dirt roads, to visit Ian's friend, Man. His house had no walls but compared to our camp out bush it was luxurious, especially as I was seven months pregnant. It hadn't rained there for ages but it had further out and the Daly, this huge, holy river which Man called the Ganges of the Territory, was all the way up. It was stunning and the bridge was under water, which meant nobody could cross it.

I was due right in the middle of the rain season, and Man was keen for the baby to be born at his place. He grew fruit and vegetables and was always putting in plumbing and water tanks. 'I know the rains will be here,' he said. 'But my neighbour's got a quad bike that will get you through anything.' So even his neighbours were in on it. But when I talked to the health worker at the clinic down there—Man had asked me to and it was the first time I'd spoken to anyone medical—she didn't want me to risk it. She told me to get myself a midwife, which was probably impossible as I was so far into the pregnancy, or talk to the hospital in Darwin.

I hadn't planned anything at all and had no idea where I'd have the baby but even though her words stayed in my head, I dismissed them. I really believed in Ian and me. We were skinny and strong. We'd travelled together from India all the way to Denmark. And I never guessed the things that could happen when travelling through Iran and Pakistan. We kept it together and looked after each other and I had faith in him. And that's what he wanted.

We spent about two weeks driving to the Daly and around Batchelor on dirt roads, bumping around in that silly old van, and I became very emotional. I got all cross with Ian and at one point decided I was going to hitch back to Darwin—which wouldn't have been easy as no trucks could get across the river. 'She's too angry,' Ian said. 'I can't do anything.' Man was really kind. 'Come on, Jenny,' he said. 'Don't be silly. I don't think you should hitch-hike anywhere, I think you should stay with us.'

I eventually calmed down and we drove Man back to his home. My back was hurting really low down and I made Ian stop the van several times along the way so I could get out and stretch by the road. He rubbed my sore spots till I felt good again and I also had read a terrific book about the Alexander technique, which gave me some good, simple exercises to do. We slept under our mosquito net in the van near Man's house and I got up twice in the night and walked around the hillside until my back felt better, saying Hail Marys and Hare Krishnas.

It was still hurting the next morning, to my complete surprise. 'Oh God,' I said to Ian. 'If these are going to go on for another month, then I've got to have some respite.' I thought some marijuana would be a nice sort of pain relief so I kissed Man goodbye and we headed north.

It was such a strange journey back to Mick's. We were sun-drying wild bananas on tin plates on the roof of the van—sun-dried bananas are incredible—but we'd always forget them. We'd drive off and suddenly say, 'The bananas!'

and have to do a U-ey and go back and look for them.

The van was overheating and I was soon lying in the back saying the rosary. 'Oh, this is intense pain,' I moaned. 'Do you think the baby's coming?' Ian asked. 'No, God,' I said. 'Another month.' I didn't think the pain had anything to do with the baby arriving.

It was a big job to get that van to Mick's place and as we pulled in, the motor conked out. Mick came out to greet us. 'Hey, you've come here to have the baby,' he said. And that was probably the last time I scoffed at the idea.

Mick took us around to show us the work he'd done over the past couple of weeks when suddenly I felt that pain again and I pulled off all my clothes and dropped to my knees and told Ian to rub my lower back. He was incredible. He acted on anything I wanted. But Mick had never seen me naked and here I was on my hands and knees with almond oil on my arse.

By mid-afternoon it had become incredibly hot, so we moved inside where the air was cooler. The house was one big round room with a sunken floor and a mattress in the middle. There was an opening for an entry on each side and a tin roof overhung the thick rock walls. It was breezy and we burnt incense to keep the sandflies and mozzies away.

Mick cooked me up some weed with wild bananas, and then drove off. The shocking cramps started to come more often and fiercely and when I started to cry Ian took me on a long meditation he made up on the moment. He talked about the colour blue and all the places we'd been. 'Imagine you are lying on your back in a big cold lake and you're looking up and what do you see?' he asked. And I said, 'I can see blue sky.' 'Are you cool in that cold blue water?'

He talked me into a trance and when Mick returned an hour or so later with his friend Kim, I was calm and greeted them with a big smile.

I didn't know Mick was bringing Kim back but we were pleased to see her. She'd had a baby, but when she turned up she said, 'Sorry guys, I had a Caesarean.' It didn't matter though because she knew about the nice things and had brought some bottles of icy water from her fridge.

The pain was intense but I was relaxed. The weed was working and I loved the company. Between contractions, I would sit on my knees on the mattress and everyone sat around telling silly stories. 'Oh, oh, please now,' I'd say when a contraction came and they'd all rush over to their positions. I was in my favourite cat pose on hands and knees. Ian's job was to rub oil on my lower back and Kim was in charge of the water. After a contraction, I'd sit back on my haunches, and they'd all flop somewhere and start cracking jokes again.

I'm sure natural endorphins were pumping through me and I was amazed. I could see my pelvis opening up and my hips were getting wider and wider. I'm quite flexible but soon my hips were touching the mattress between my heels. It looked bizarre.

I still felt that the baby should stay in—it was just too early—so I tried to stay as horizontal as possible. I was on my hands and knees and had my bottom end in the air during the contractions so there was no gravity, but when my waters broke at sunset, I knew the baby was going to come soon and I started to get excited.

Kim had called the Darwin hospital from her place—I suspect she said something like, 'Emergency. There's a lady having a baby out bush'—and the hospital chartered a ferry and sent a team across the harbour. I hadn't asked for that at all but when Kim handed me her mobile and the doctor, who was on her way, started asking me questions, I was as polite as could be. 'Yes, it hurts a lot,' I shouted down the line. 'Yes. I think the baby is coming.' I wasn't in a state to speak, so I was yelling while Badger, Mick's scruffy rust and brown-coloured cattle dog, barked away outside.

There was no electricity, not even any lines nearby, so as night came candles were lit and I heard my hips creaking. The baby wasn't pushing but seemed to have moved into position so I didn't sit back on my knees again. 'I can see the baby's head,' said Ian. 'Just push and it will come out.'

Mick held my arms and I pushed only once, and there was a great whoosh, whoosh. It was the most beautiful, gorgeous feeling, and Pandy came out just as the big full moon was rising.

Mick had his hands on my belly and later said he felt it just disappear. Ian was behind me and the baby just slipped into his arms and he held her. Then I heard whispering. The umbilical cord seemed to be very long and wrapped all around, so they gently weaved her back in and out to untangle her. And that's when Kim, who had been wonderful, became super-useful. 'Give her to her mum,' she said. I sat up against a post and they gave my baby to me. *Oh, beautiful, beautiful*, I thought. 'Put her on your breast,' Kim said. And I did and Pandy started sucking straight away: no hesitation. By candlelight, her eyes were open wide, looking all around.

She came out beautifully. She was small—probably less than five pounds—and strong and alert. Incredibly, she seemed able to hold her head up. It was the right time for her and she was such a little beauty.

Badger was still having a bit of a woof, so Mick went outside and made a fuss of her and then he was back teasing me.

He and Ian wanted to cut the cord. 'What's the rush?' I asked and told them to wait for the placenta. And 20 minutes later I felt this clunk, clunk, so I leant forward on my knees and the placenta whooshed through, easy as can be.

I'd remembered from high school first aid that the umbilical cord should be tied in three places before snipping between the second and the third tie. So Mick offered a clean T-shirt and ripped it into strips and they tied the cord. They only did it in two places—I wasn't watching—and used scissors boiled and rinsed in tea tree oil. They left about 25 centimetres attached to her belly button.

The doctor and paramedic arrived shortly afterwards with their equipment, including a humidicrib, but nothing was brought out of the car. 'Wow, I've never seen anything like this before,' said the paramedic, a sweet-voiced older woman. 'Congratulations.' The doctor was also pleased. She asked me a few questions and gave the baby a thorough look. 'It's a really healthy little bub,' she said. She and Ian had a close look at the placenta to make sure none of it was left inside, but they didn't stay long. There really was no need.

I was incredibly sweaty and rinsed myself under the tap at the water tank. The boys wanted to wash little Pandy and I let them. They washed her very gently, especially around her head, which was so soft. It still had blood on it a few days later when Badger, who once had a litter of puppies, came and licked it all off. A rough tongue really was the perfect thing for a soft fontanelle.

That noisy van never did start again. We pushed it into a grove of trees a few days later and put up a tarp for shade and made it cool and cosy and we lived there for the next six months with trips into Darwin.

The rains came and made life easy and it was a brilliant time. My mother and sister sent snowy-white nappies that washed clean in a bucket and several times a day I'd sit in a 44-gallon drum full of fresh rainwater, often holding Pandy. Every fortnight someone would go to town for supplies and one day a carload of Belyuen people came to see the baby, which was an honour as she had been born on their land and came out so strong.

I tried to be out bush for the birth of my second baby four years later, but it didn't quite work out that way. We'd come home to Darwin after an incredible year in Amsterdam, where I worked as a musician, artist and waitress. Most births in The Netherlands were home births, but I longed for the tropics, and so did Pandy.

We lived with my great friend Surabhi Dasi at the Hari Krishna temple in Stuart Park. I loved the company of Surabhi's children and grandchildren and the house was often filled with guests. We slept out on a big covered balcony, surrounded by palm trees. I was too tired for exercise this time so I would ride my bicycle around the suburbs to relax.

Incredibly, Mick now lived around the corner and one

night Ian and I rode around to see him, with me sitting on the handlebars. My belly was huge and I laughed so much I wet my pants.

But there wasn't much I found funny when the birth day came for my second child. Two weeks away from the baby's due date in March 2002, I woke up at 8 a.m. in intense pain and got straight under the shower. I ran the water so hot my skin burned, but I needed it for the pain in my back.

I was too agitated to dress and began pacing around the balcony giving orders. Cedar, a friend downstairs, called up, 'Is there anything I can do?' 'Yes, come on up,' I yelled back and I soon had her at work. Surabhi's job was to fill a bucket with hot water for the stack of cloth nappies I'd bought and she also made me fresh hibiscus tea to make me slippery and fenugreek tea to ease my cramps. Cedar held a hot, wet nappy under my belly and Ian rubbed oil into the base of my back. I was drinking hot drinks rather than cold ones this time and found them very comforting.

Pandy sat in a beanbag about four feet away from me through the whole birth, with her backpack on. She was so cute and would sometimes creep forward to put ice in my mouth. But it was a shame no one had thought to walk her next door to my neighbour, who would have taken great care of her. There was just no time.

I wasn't in that serene state of mind like last time. There was no relaxing between contractions, even for Ian, and I really wondered where my endorphins were as it was so much more painful. 'The baby's crowning,' said Surabhi less than an hour after I'd woken up. He was obviously a chunky bubba and his big head had been poking between my legs for the last ten minutes. I was terrified of a big tear, but he wouldn't wait. Freddy pushed his way through—he couldn't have come out any faster—and I knew from the sting that I had ripped at the side.

He was a really nice golden brown colour, but I was in such a daze that I just kept on saying how sore I was. Freddy kept his eyes shut, except for the occasional squinty glance, and was still grumbling at midnight.

Pandy says she wants babies but also says she doesn't because they hurt. I can understand that after what she saw, but I love telling Pandy the story of her birth. 'You were born when the full moon was rising,' I say, and she cuddles in close. She particularly loves the part where Badger licks the blood off her head.

Birth for me has never been a nightmare. It doesn't need to be. My own birth was pretty straightforward with my father there, catching me, and I love it that my babies came out strong and were caught by their dad. I feel very lucky and give full credit to the gods and angels, especially Mary.

Postscript

At her family's urging, Jenny went to a doctor for a check-up a few weeks after her daughter's birth. The reaction was decidedly icy. 'The doctor was like, "If you're going to do things without the medical profession, don't expect us to help you",' says Jenny. But the visit served its purpose. 'I was able to say to my mum that I'd been,' she says.

Today, she lives in New South Wales in a house without mains power but with a phone line, and a forest and a donkey out back. 'Pandy loves her friends and relations and her favourite subjects at school are soccer and scripture,' says Jenny who changed some names for this story. 'Freddy likes bicycles and helmets and most afternoons will push his favourite chickens round in a pram.'

Ian works at a school, mostly teaching music, and runs an event production company. His band plays at children's concerts, outdoor events and all-night dance parties. And Jenny, who grew up in a big bustling family with cousins around the corner, isn't giving up on the idea of more children. 'I would like a whole tribe of them,' she says. 'Healthy bubbas—they're the best thing in the world.'

The perfect family

PENNY McCARTHY

I cried when I found out I was pregnant in 1995 at the age of 26—and they weren't tears of joy. I knew I'd have kids one day but falling pregnant really was the furthermost thing from my mind. I had just started the fashion editor job I'd always wanted, I was living with Brendan, going out to a party every weekend, and although I wasn't that young, it seemed it.

But it wasn't long before I started getting really excited about being pregnant. My parents were thrilled and Brendan was over the moon. He's one of six kids and when I'd met him two years earlier he'd told me he wanted six of his own. He was clucky from the age of about 22 and was very much into family. I'd always found that very appealing about him.

A lot of my friends and people at work were shocked. I think they thought, *God, how's Penny, the career-slash-party girl going to do this?* And all I heard were negatives about how hard it was going to be. 'Just wait, just wait,' people would say.

I felt really good throughout the pregnancy. I worked up until 38 weeks, was on 5 a.m. fashion shoots and caught the bus to work. I had so much energy, which probably had a lot to do with my age.

But I knew nothing about babies. We went to the pre-natal class and saw that lovely seventies video of a woman giving birth and I thought, *Oh my God, this just doesn't look human.* It really did look strange and revolting when you'd never seen it before, but I wasn't too concerned. I knew I was in good hands.

On 22 May 1996, I went for a very long walk with a friend around Paddington. I came home, sat down with Brendan at 8.30 p.m. to watch *Melrose Place* and started to get a couple of subtle little twinges. I didn't say anything at first, but then I had another one. 'I think something's happening,' I told Brendan.

I went upstairs and sat on the toilet and my waters broke. Stupidly, I panicked and thought it was part of the baby. 'Brendan, something's fallen in the toilet,' I shouted to him. 'That's your mucus plug, dear,' he replied, in the middle of a phone call with the hospital. 'It's all right.' I was very, very naive. And then we got into bed and cuddled.

The contractions started getting really severe around midnight, so I called Mum and she came and picked us up. By the time we arrived at the hospital it was one o'clock and I was well on the way, about three or four centimetres dilated. There was no massaging or music. I was feeling awful and vomited a few times. I curled up on the bed like a little animal, moaning and groaning. I was in so much pain I thought I was going to black out.

I really had no birth plan and at about three o'clock one

of the nurses asked if I wanted an epidural. 'What do you think?' I asked Mum. 'Darling,' she said, 'there are no medals for not having one.'

Brendan left the room—he faints when he has needles himself—and I had the epidural and it was lovely. I was relaxed and calm. I wasn't in that mad rage any more and I felt I could really enjoy the whole birth.

I couldn't believe it when I finally pushed Ruby out at sunrise. 'Look, it's a baby,' I said. I don't know what I was expecting, an octopus or something, but there was this beautiful, big, whole baby and I was absolutely blown away. I felt so clever.

And the minute I held her, I thought, *What on earth was everyone talking about? This is the best thing in the world.* I didn't want to put her down and Brendan had a grin from ear to ear for a week.

I had a contract with my magazine and another woman there, who'd already had two babies, told me I'd be bored by six months and would definitely want to go back to work. But I started getting panicky when four months came around. *I can't leave this baby and go back to work,* I thought. *What could be more important than being home with her?* So I never went back.

I loved being a mother. It was fantastic and so much fun. I never missed my old life. I was doing what I loved. And after Ruby was born, I definitely knew I wanted a large family.

Brendan and I were married in February 1997 when Ruby was eight months old. Ruby was the flower-girl and it was very special. Not long after, we moved to Geneva for Brendan's work and I became pregnant again, but I didn't know until I was about nine weeks. I'd done a pregnancy test but it was in German and I couldn't read it: I thought it said negative. So there I was in Paris drinking away, wondering why I was so tired. My gums started to bleed and that's when I knew I was pregnant.

We soon moved back to Australia and I had a very easy pregnancy. I woke up in labour on 11 March 1998, went shopping for a camera, had a few doughnuts and went to the hospital. I was handling the contractions okay. *This isn't that bad*, I thought, *maybe I can do it*. But then it all turned around so fast and hit me. 'Oh no, here we go again,' I said, 'now I remember.' And I asked for an epidural.

It was a slow process pushing out this baby—he had a bigger head than Ruby—but when Jimmy arrived, I was instantly in love again.

It was a very straightforward birth. I was calm and enjoyed it. I had Rhesus-negative blood and both my babies had Rhesus-positive blood, so I had to be injected with anti-D immunoglobulin after the births. It was basically to make sure I didn't build up any antibodies in my system that could damage any future babies, but there wasn't any drama.

We really had the perfect life. Brendan was busy working in finance, we were renovating our home and we had these two beautiful babies under two. I cherished every day and never wished it away. By the time Jimmy was one, I wanted another little baby again, so at 30 I became pregnant with our third child while most of my friends were still thinking about their first.

My GP confirmed the pregnancy and told me about the new nuchal translucency test, which measured the fluid at the back of a baby's neck and was supposed to be an indicator for Down syndrome. It hadn't been around for my other two babies and although my GP didn't recommend it—she thought it made people paranoid—I jumped at the chance to see the baby.

I went to have the ultrasound when I was about 12 weeks and it took a very long time. 'Is everything all right?' I asked. 'Yes, yes,' said the technician. 'The baby's in a funny position, we need to get a better view.' She did an internal ultrasound as well.

The doctor came in to give me the results. 'Your chances have increased,' he said, and my heart started racing. 'Is something wrong with my baby?' I asked, and he explained that after taking into account my age and the results of the test, which showed more fluid than usual, my chances of having a Down syndrome baby were now one in 426. The cut-off for concern was one in 250, so I was still in what's classified as the normal range.

I left the doctor's office and didn't feel right. I read the report again and called my obstetrician. 'I've got a very high chance of having a baby with Down syndrome,' I said. He asked how old I was and I told him. 'Nope,' he said. 'You've got two perfect children, this is your third child and you're not in that category.' I was young and age was obviously on my side.

The nuchal test was new, not many people had had it and the doctors were saying it was a 'soft indicator'. I didn't have it with the other two and I really didn't know what to go by.

'Darl, what if the baby's got Down syndrome?' I asked Brendan later. 'Well,' he said, 'what are we going to do about it? The baby's in there from the beginning.' I thought about having an amniocentesis, but I knew we'd never have done anything: I don't think Brendan would have ever terminated a pregnancy. He was adamant, more so than me, and I think he swayed me a little bit. So in the end I thought, *Well, I'm not going to jeopardise this baby I'm carrying.* And that was it and I never really thought about it again.

Shortly after this, my obstetrician called and told me Rhesus antibodies had shown up in my blood tests. Some of Jimmy's blood must have remained in my body after his birth even though I'd had the anti-D injection. And the antibodies could be really dangerous: my unborn baby's blood would fight the antibodies and it was at risk of being severely anaemic. In very bad cases, the baby could go into cardiac arrest and die.

It was a mystery how I'd gotten it. I looked back at my records and although I was given the injection before the 72-hour cut-off, it was close to it. And apparently one per cent of women require a second injection. I must have needed one but my blood hadn't been checked.

My obstetrician was very reassuring though. He told me the baby would probably need to be delivered a week or so early to be safe and my blood needed to be checked constantly to see where my levels were. He said if the level got above four it was really dangerous, but throughout the pregnancy everything seemed fine and the levels remained low. I felt good, I was carrying the baby in the same way I had with the other two and the 18-week scan showed that all was fine: size, dates, everything.

My obstetrician went on holidays late in the pregnancy and I was due to see his stand-in for my 37-week check.

I nearly didn't go. *Oh, third baby,* I thought. *I can't be bothered.* But I did, and when I asked the stand-in, who I'd never met before, what the antibody level was, he said, very calmly: 'Eight-point-two.' 'Oh my God,' I said, and started crying hysterically. I immediately thought the baby was going to die. He went to speak to the paediatrician and came back into the office a few minutes later. 'Go home and pack,' he said. 'You've got to be induced immediately.'

I was in an absolute state. I saw the paediatrician, called Brendan and went home and packed, and my mother came and took Ruby and Jimmy. I was so upset and worried. My doctor wasn't there, some doctor I didn't know was in charge and I felt totally out of control.

Brendan and I went to the hospital. The doctor had said I was already two centimetres dilated during that day's examination and before the midwife put the gel on to my cervix to induce me, she checked the baby. 'Oh my gosh,' she said. 'I can't tell where this baby's head is. If it's breech, I can't induce you.' But she found it, and they put the gel on at three o'clock in the morning.

Nothing was happening, so they broke my waters at seven with the knitting needles. That got the labour going and I had the epidural straight away.

Brendan stayed calm and read the newspaper and we talked about names—Billy or Max if the baby was a boy. They were monitoring the baby and it seemed to be in great condition, but I was incredibly nervous. I was trying to keep it together but all I really wanted to do was get the baby out and make sure everything was fine.

No one was giving anything away about what was

going to happen—I don't think my doctor wanted to distress me any more than I already was—but they did say the best-case scenario would be that the baby would be jaundiced and need some lights. The worst, he would need a blood transfusion.

Eventually it came time to push. It was an easy delivery and when I pushed out the head, my obstetrician said, 'I think this one's a girl. It looks very pretty.' But when the baby came out, he said, 'No, no. It's a boy.'

I was thrilled and I looked down and thought that he didn't look like the other babies. He was three weeks early, so he was smaller, and he did look pretty—he had this little delicate face with much smaller features and these little eyes. I called my mum. 'It's a boy!' I said. 'He looks like me when I was born. He's got little Chinese eyes.'

They took him away to inspect him and then they gave him to me for a cuddle and I put him to my bosom. I could see he was starting to turn yellow and they took him away again. My sister Sally had just arrived and went over to where the nurses, doctor and paediatrician were huddled around a table with lights on him. They were very quiet and as Sally went to stand beside them, they kind of elbowed her out of the way and took him to another room.

Minutes later, they came back in and I saw this look on the paediatrician's face. I thought, *Oh God, he hasn't died, has he?* I looked at his lips and somehow I knew what he was going to say. 'Your little boy has Down syndrome,' he said. The words sounded like they were on this sort of weird, foggy loudspeaker. It was as if I had just been told, 'Your husband's died in a car crash.'

Brendan started crying straight away and apparently I started talking. 'It doesn't matter,' I said. 'It doesn't matter. It's all right. It doesn't matter. We've still got a baby, he's going to be beautiful.' Me, the eternal optimist.

They brought him in and I cuddled him. I had to call my parents back, and I asked them to sit down before I told them. I was in shock and felt like I was dreaming. The baby was now as orange as a pumpkin and someone said, 'We have to take him away. We think he's going to need a blood transfusion.'

And so the nightmare began. They took him to intensive care and I returned to the maternity ward without my baby. And if ever I needed to have a baby to cuddle and bond with, he was the one.

Just before they started the transfusion—they had to do it as soon as possible—the doctor came and told me that Max had a little hole in his heart. 'We have to tell you, the blood transfusion puts a lot of pressure on his heart,' the doctor said. And that was the final straw. Mum and Dad were in the room by then and I started crying for the first time. 'Could anything else go wrong?' I said. 'Oh God, this poor little boy. It's not fair. How could this happen? What's gone wrong?'

I went down to intensive care and watched my newborn baby boy have a blood transfusion later that night. It was such a slow process—they put in one cannula of blood and took one out—and there were four doctors standing around him. I stood there in a state of shock and thought, *How could I have this Down syndrome baby having a blood transfusion? This is not my life. This happens to other people, not me.* As a mother your worst nightmare is that there's something wrong with the baby. And this was my worst nightmare.

Brendan stayed with me in hospital but I couldn't sleep. I kept thinking it was a dream, that it wasn't real. They gave me sleeping pills and for the first four nights I'd wake up in the morning and for that split second think, *Oh my God. Is it true?* And then I'd remember, no, it's not a dream. It's still here.

I was in tears for most of the time in hospital and was numb. Absolutely numb. I went to the special care nursery one night and a girl I went to school with was there. 'I think we're in the same boat,' she said, but I wasn't in the mood to chat. 'What do you mean?' I asked. 'My little boy has Down syndrome, too,' she said. I couldn't believe it and neither could the hospital. They had three Down syndrome babies born within three days to mothers all under 35. Normally they had one a year.

It was such a confusing time. Sometimes I'd think, *Oh God, snap out of it, it's not that bad.* And then I'd think, *Yes it is.* And I'd fantasise about the weirdest things. At one point I thought, *Maybe it's better if he dies. I can walk out of here and pretend none of this has ever happened and I will go home and have another baby.* And then I'd go down to intensive care and see this poor baby lying there and think, *Oh God, please don't die. Please don't die.* There could not have been anything worse. I was still trying to get my head around everything but that maternal thing was stronger than anything else.

But it was a sad sort of maternal feeling, not a joyous one. The doctors were asking me if I was touching him. I couldn't pick him up for the first five days but of course

I was touching him. I didn't feel cold towards him and I don't think I could: he was my baby, he'd been inside me for eight months, he was my own flesh and blood. But I didn't feel as in love as I was with the other two and sometimes I went through the motions of it all and really felt nothing. Maybe that's how women feel when they don't bond with their babies. I hadn't felt like that before and that's what made me sad.

It was so hard trying to get my head around that it was forever. Sometimes I'd think, *If only he'd had bloody cancer or something that could be cured*. I thought it was going to ruin all our lives, especially Ruby's and Jimmy's, and I thought I'd never smile again. I worried about his future. I didn't know what was going to happen or how he was going to turn out. It was a fear of the unknown.

And it was so horrible to be in that hospital room without my baby by my side. I felt like I hadn't even had a baby, let alone one with Down syndrome. I felt so ripped off. Having a baby is supposed to be the best moment of your life and it had turned into the worst. There was no joy and no elation.

Sally told a lot of people, but there were no visitors. There was nothing to see as the baby was in intensive care, and people didn't know how to react. Some didn't contact me, which was the most dreadful thing as I'd just had a baby above all else, but my good friends were incredible. I received the most beautiful letter from a very good friend the day after Max was born. 'No matter what,' he wrote, 'Max is a McCarthy. All your children are beautiful and he will be no different.' Brendan's dad was the first person to ring up and say 'Congratulations. Congratulations on your beautiful boy', which made us both cry.

Brendan was incredible. He couldn't have handled it better. He was sad but not overly sad, and he loved and bonded with Max straight away. He was very strong and was like, 'It's all right. This is just the way it is.' He was fine with it all after a couple of months and, I admit, moved on a lot faster than I did. They say the chances of splitting up are far greater for couples that have children with special needs, but it went the other way for us. It bonded us together and we felt very close through the whole thing.

After four days in hospital I said, 'I've got to get out of here', and left without my baby. I couldn't stand it in there any longer. I was desperate to get Max home, breastfeed him, cluck around him and get him dressed in his own clothes and into his own little bed, but he needed to stay in hospital for another ten days. That had nothing to do with the Down's, it was all to do with Rhesus disease. He came home on 23 December 1999, just in time for Christmas.

The first few months were very up and down. Sometimes I felt fine, other times I just wanted to cry. I was having dreadful panic attacks, thinking that something was going to happen to Ruby and Jimmy, but it was probably those two who got me through it. They were such a good distraction and it was hard to be depressed when you've got these two beautiful healthy kids running around. I didn't want them to think, *Why is Mummy upset?* So I tried to hide it and used to cry in the shower a lot and in the car.

I blamed myself for a long time after Max's birth. I felt like my body had failed me. I'd think, *Why did my body do* this? Why didn't the cells align properly? Did I drink when I was pregnant? What if I hadn't had sex that night? I felt sorry this poor little child was going to lead a hard life because of me. It certainly wasn't his fault, it wasn't the doctor's fault. The baby was like that in the beginning. But the doctors told me there was nothing I had done for Max to have Down syndrome.

I never dwelt on the fact that we hadn't found out earlier. Would we have terminated? Could I have lived with myself for doing that? I don't think so. I would have felt incredibly weak doing that just because the child wasn't perfect. But there is no way in the world I would have done anything if I'd known what Max would be like today.

After Max came home, I was obsessed with finding out what the future held and wanted to meet other families and find out what other children were like. I was really curious and when I did meet people, it was a big relief. And a great support. Other mothers with Down syndrome children were the only people who really understood what it was like in those early days.

I read a lot of literature and found it so depressing. It painted the worst possible picture and I stopped reading it after a while. I realised a lot of the stuff didn't apply to Max—the hole in his heart had closed over and he was so healthy—and I decided I would do my own thing and raise him the way I'd raised my other children.

The other kids loved Max immediately and our families and friends all adored him and clucked over him, which was really important to us. Everyone was really accepting and just got used to the way it was.

It probably took about eight months before I didn't feel the grief and sadness I had felt after his birth. Time heals, but it took a long time, and I didn't enjoy him being a baby. Babies are supposed to be gorgeous and perfect and Max was never the perfect baby. But it really wasn't until he was two that I completely stopped thinking, *Oh, imagine if he was normal*. By then I was madly in love with him and didn't think of him in terms of Down syndrome. But I definitely think the final healing process was having another baby.

I knew I would have another child from the day Max was born. My obstetrician had told me it was probably unlikely I could have more children because of the Rhesus disease—it gets worse with each baby—but I was determined. I didn't want Max to be the youngest child. I thought another child would be fantastic for his development, and I'd always wanted four children—at least. But there were going to be risks.

Everyone thought I was mad doing it again. A lot of people were worried about the Down syndrome thing, but that was never our concern. The Rhesus disease was always our concern.

I went to see the head of obstetrics at one hospital and he was incredibly negative. 'What sex are your children?' he asked. When I told him, he said, 'Well, you've got both.' I couldn't see what that had to do with anything, and he also made a comment about my chances of having another Down syndrome baby.

I couldn't stand to be told I wasn't allowed to have as many children as I wanted, particularly after Max. So I shopped around. Eventually I found an amazing woman who specialised in Rhesus disease and I had my files sent to her. She was very positive and told me that if I fell pregnant, I'd get to about 34 weeks and would need to have the baby then. I already had one special needs child, so to have a very premature baby was a concern to me, but she said the outcome would be very good. She told me there might be short-term feeding problems and the baby would need to be kept warm, but there would be no long-term effects of prematurity.

I knew what I was in for but I so wanted to have another baby, and in early 2002 I fell pregnant with our fourth baby and the pregnancy was classified as high risk. The nuchal translucency looked good this time and everything else was fantastic, but because I'd already had a baby with Down syndrome my chance of having another was one in 100.

It was a very difficult decision for me to have an amnio. I knew that if I miscarried, I probably wouldn't be able to have another pregnancy because of the Rhesus problem, and I ended up putting it off until week 17, when the niggling in the back of my mind just got the better of me. But the results were fine, although the amnio confirmed the baby had a different blood type to mine, so I was monitored very closely—weekly ultrasounds from week 22 and blood tests every week.

I was very anxious—I once went in for a test because I couldn't feel the baby moving—but besides a heavy bleed early in the pregnancy, everything went well. The hospital was graphing my levels and every week my doctor said, 'This is incredible.'

And then, at my 34-week ultrasound, my levels went boom, just as my doctor had predicted. 'Okay, you'd better go home,' she said. 'The baby's fine now but we want to get it out, healthy and in a good condition. I'll book you in for tomorrow.' The baby was becoming anaemic and they were trying to avoid a blood transfusion.

The next day I was back in hospital having a steroid injection to help strengthen the baby's lungs and I was induced the following morning with the gel. But my body just wasn't ready. Everything was slow and haphazard, and by mid-morning they were pumping the syntocinon drip into me to try and get me to labour. My cervix was still right back and the doctor eventually came in and ripped it forward. That was brutal.

I was so anxious throughout the labour, particularly after Max's birth. I wanted everything to hurry up but my cervix wouldn't dilate and although the baby was never distressed, I almost said, 'Just do a Caesarean.' It wasn't a happy, lovey-dovey birth experience by any means. I was in it for the baby, not the birth, and all I was thinking about was getting that baby out.

Finally, just before 10 p.m. the time came to push—and there wasn't much pushing because the baby was so tiny. The doctor had said it would be a good sign if the baby came out crying, and Ava came out kicking and screaming and looking pink. She was so small—five pounds—but she was perfectly formed. She was like one of those little Baby Bjorn dolls. She was so sweet, but the labour was 15 hours and the whole experience was definitely the worst of the lot.

I was so relieved and happy with my little girl, but after a couple of days I could see her starting to go yellow. And on day three, the doctor came and told me Ava would need a blood transfusion. 'Is there any risk?' I asked, in tears. 'I can't lie to you,' the doctor said. 'There is a risk. She's a six-week premature baby having a major blood transfusion and we don't know how she's going to react to the new blood.'

I was distraught. I really thought I'd been through enough. Mum and I watched them set up the equipment in intensive care, but I had to leave. I was so close to getting her and started feeling superstitious that something would go wrong.

But it didn't. She remained in intensive care for a few days and was in hospital for three weeks over Christmas. I was expressing milk eight times a day, because it was virtually impossible to feed her. She just wouldn't attach. But she was healthy—they called her the disco queen because she'd come alive at night—and today you'd never know she'd been premature.

I had two babies that were easy and two that were a struggle to get here. I look back on the time I had Max and it really was the worst period of my life—there was so much grief—but I just don't apply any of that to the child he is today. I can't look at him and feel sad. I absolutely adore him. He's a fun, cheeky, happy, loving, gorgeous little boy and I can't imagine our life without him.

I do feel frustrated with Max at times—everything happens a lot slower and you've got to put more effort into things—but I get frustrated with all my kids at some point. There's a side to our family that wasn't there before and Max has given an extra depth to all of us.

I always used to think, *Imagine if he was just normal.* Now I think, *My God, what if he wasn't the way he was?* It's like saying, 'Suppose Ruby was a boy?' I couldn't imagine him not being the way he is. I'd miss it—those little sausage fingers and soft little skin. Max is just how he was meant to be. Once I thought I had the perfect family life, which was no longer perfect. I don't feel like that now because I have got the perfect family. I feel incredibly blessed.

Postscript

From the day Penny McCarthy and Brendan took Max home from hospital, he has been treated as one of the brood. 'We're not trivialising his disability,' she says, 'but we've certainly made no exceptions for him. He's been treated just like one of the other kids and always will be.'

Max had to have physiotherapy for the first couple of years of his life—he didn't walk until he was two and a half—and has speech therapy twice a week. His comprehension is good, says Penny, but his speech is 'a lot slower than I thought it would be'.

Today, Max is a skilled trampoliner and keen swimmer (with a bubble) and goes to the same preschool his older brother, Jimmy, and older sister, Ruby, went to. He is due to start school in 2006. 'I think the most important thing to us was that he would be able to blend in and be one of the kids,' says Penny, 'and that's never been a problem. It's been very easy for him and he's loved it.'

While she says she occasionally wonders how Ruby, Jimmy and Ava will manage with Max once she and Brendan are gone—'You think of everything,' she says—she looks forward to Max's future without any of the sadness she once had. 'It's just like with other kids, what's the next stage for him,' she says.

And despite her last two difficult births, Penny says she would have another baby if she could. 'I can't now, but I still would have had five,' she says. 'Four has never felt like that many. But four is a good number. Definitely a good number.'

Mascot for a nation

KIRSTY SWORD GUSMÃO

Even though I was in my early thirties by the time Xanana and I were able to begin life together as a relatively normal couple, I wasn't sure that becoming a mother was my cup of tea. Between 1999 and 2001 I was virtually Xanana's sole support person, who was then working towards rebuilding East Timor, and was rather overwhelmed by my responsibilities. I didn't have a lot of time to contemplate whether or not I had any maternal instincts.

Xanana and I had earlier entertained some fanciful dreams of becoming parents during his years as the jailed leader of the East Timorese resistance movement, and had sometimes bemoaned that our circumstances made my becoming pregnant an impossibility. We had only met face to face twice between 1994 and 1998—and then under the close watch of prison guards.

Sometime in August 1994, Xanana had a consultation with a fellow inmate at Cipinang High Security Prison in East Jakarta who was a bit of a soothsayer or fortune-teller.

During their conversation and palm reading, Xanana asked the man whether or not he would remarry and have more children. The answer on both scores was 'yes', something which caused Xanana to shout out with glee.

When Xanana insisted upon knowing how many children he would father, the answer was, 'Two or three.' Who knows whether it was the prospect of having more children or the fortune-teller's other predictions that Xanana would live to a ripe old age and find happiness in his fifties and sixties which caused him to hum to himself as he returned to his cell.

What nobody could have foreseen back then was the extraordinary series of political developments within Indonesia which would alter the course of East Timor's fate and indeed my own.

In May 1998, President Suharto stepped down after 30 years at the helm in Indonesia amid calls for reform and democratisation. His successor, President B.J. Habibie, sanctioned the holding of a 'popular consultation' to determine the future of East Timor. In February 1999, Xanana was released from Cipinang, although he remained under house arrest in Jakarta, and on 30 August 1999, 78.5 per cent of East Timorese voted to 'separate' from Indonesia. The violence and systematic destruction of public and private property which followed meant that the months afterwards were ones of hard work and emotional pain for Xanana and me.

On 7 September 1999, Xanana was finally given his freedom, and in early January 2000 we took a brief but sorely needed holiday on the Mornington Peninsula in Victoria. It was the first chance we'd had the time to focus on ourselves for more than a year and it was then that we conceived our first child.

Later that month, we were visiting a number of Asian capitals with Dr Jose Ramos-Horta and two UN staffers and, between official meetings and duties, I bought a home pregnancy testing kit at a pharmacy in a crowded Singapore shopping mall. But it wasn't until we reached Manila a few days later that I had the peace of mind—and the courage—to do the test.

For the sake of propriety, Xanana and I were in separate rooms of the plush Manila Hotel—we were not married, and Xanana had had little time to devote to the question of filing for divorce from his first wife, although the process was in motion. I did the test in the bathroom of Xanana's suite and didn't know whether to laugh or cry when it showed a positive result.

Xanana's reaction was not what I had hoped. 'I am not sure that now is the right time,' he said. I was hurt and disappointed and shortly afterwards returned to my own room, overcome by sadness and physical exhaustion. We'd been keeping a heavy schedule, and by now my body was reacting to the early stages of pregnancy.

But, less than an hour later, Xanana called me back to his room and now there was a gleam of excitement in his eye. He'd had time to digest the news and was delighted about the prospects of being a father again. It seemed that things were going to be okay after all.

Somehow I managed to find the time to read up on the stages of pregnancy amid the official engagements and busy schedule we kept in the following months. In March I passed up the opportunity to visit the Nordic countries and Africa with Xanana in order to travel to Melbourne where I had my first antenatal check-up and ultrasound at the Royal Women's Hospital. The little creature swimming deep in my belly looked more like a restless shellfish than a baby, and that afternoon my mother and I replayed the video image over and over again in her Northcote flat.

I felt both elated and a little anxious. I didn't know anything about the availability of antenatal care in Dili. The East Timorese people had welcomed me to date, but how would they respond once they knew I was carrying their leader's child?

I couldn't dwell on these problems when I returned to Dili. Xanana's political work, my support of him and my decision to establish Dili's first public library in the form of the Xanana Gusmão Reading Room occupied all of my time.

In April we began to break the news of my pregnancy to close friends and family. While our not being married didn't seem to cause any particular backlash, we both felt that the time was ripe to put the official stamp on our relationship, before the baby arrived in late September.

So in late May we made some tentative preparations for our marriage, and around the same time I paid my first visit to Dili National Hospital, which was being managed by the International Committee of the Red Cross. It was a far cry from the average Australian hospital but the former Dili Public Hospital was the best-equipped medical facility in the country and, surprisingly, had been spared the ravages of the militia violence of late 1999.

I had been given the names of an Irish midwife, Teresa, and her most senior East Timorese colleague, Etelvina, and they gave me a tour of the spartan maternity ward. It had a long row of delivery beds, each separated by a length of blue curtain, and a small air-conditioned consultation cubicle. Opposite was a 'safe room' set up by the UN Population Fund and a group of local non-government organisations, so rape and sexual assault victims could be examined in safety and privacy. A simple altar featuring an almost fluorescent pink and blue figurine of the Virgin Mary and a circle of lit candles sat outside the delivery rooms.

During the visit I was told about the standard antenatal care and birthing practices and I learned that although there was pain relief available in the form of pethidine, very few East Timorese women used drugs during labour. Teresa also assured me that while there was no obstetrician on staff at the hospital, her East Timorese colleagues were all highly experienced and skilled and there were foreign surgeons on hand to perform Caesarean sections, if required.

My mother, Rosalie, visited the hospital with me, a month or so later, and I soon decided that provided my pregnancy continued to be an uncomplicated one, I should give birth in Dili.

I had given serious thought to other options, including the Royal Darwin Hospital, but I wasn't comfortable with the idea of having to spend at least one month before the birth alone in Darwin, where I had few friends and no family. The chances of Xanana being able to be with me for the birth if I were to have the baby outside Timor-Leste were slim. And in any case, I really felt that I wanted my first child to be born on East Timorese soil, in the country which would be his or her home.

Teresa was extremely likeable. She had a professional air and an endearing sense of humour. She and Etelvina took joint responsibility for my antenatal care in the months that followed and I never once had any misgivings about my decision. I felt healthy, had a good diet and had no reason to believe that the birth of my first baby would be particularly difficult or dangerous.

During our monthly sessions, Teresa listened to the routine questions of a first-time mother-to-be and shared with me some of the trials she'd experienced as a foreign midwife in East Timor. She told me about the challenge of training the East Timorese midwives, as there was a definite pecking order: her midwife colleagues happily took advice and instruction from doctors and obstetricians, but didn't appreciate being lectured to by other midwives, no matter what their origin or prior experience was.

Xanana and I were married in early July, and my bump was a prominent feature of our wedding photos, as was the *tais* (length of traditional woven cloth) outfit I selected as my wedding dress. The simple Catholic ceremony in the Dare chapel in the hills south of Dili was attended by a handful of close friends, Xanana's family, my mother and my uncle (my father had died in 1988).

We took a week-long visit to New Zealand afterwards, which was mistaken by many as a honeymoon. It was a semi-official visit which, although enjoyable, involved a considerable amount of work for me as I continued to be something of a private secretary to Xanana. Maternity leave was a nice concept but a vain hope in our circumstances.

When I returned home I still managed to indulge the nesting urge as my due date approached. I decked out a corner of our bedroom with nursery gear comprising a cot, blue curtains—an ultrasound performed at Royal Darwin Hospital had revealed our baby to be a boy—colourful mobiles and a tray stacked with baby accoutrements.

Xanana returned from official visits to Portugal and Mozambique laden down by gifts of baby clothes, bed linen and toys, and I spent the final weeks of waiting arranging and re-arranging them in the few small spaces available in our somewhat baby-unfriendly home. Most importantly, by late September I had fitted flywire screens to most of the windows to keep the incessant hordes of mosquitoes to a minimum.

The six or so Brazilian bodyguards who were responsible for our security at the time seemed as nervous and anxious as we were about the imminent arrival of our baby. My mother, who had arrived in early September in anticipation of the birth of her third grandchild, came with me to my final antenatal check-ups at Dili Hospital where, somewhat to my embarrassment, the safe room had been given a fresh coat of paint and decorated with a vase of fresh frangipani and bougainvillea ahead of my expected delivery date. It was the most private area of the maternity ward and therefore considered the most appropriate space for me to give birth in.

On 30 September 2000, I woke at 1 a.m. to discover that I was alone in bed: Xanana had fallen asleep on the couch in front of the TV again. As I hauled myself upright to retrieve him, a gush of water escaped from between my legs and didn't stop until I reached the living room. I was overtaken by a mixture of excitement and pure panic.

'*A agua està a sair!* (The waters have broken!)' I shouted, and Xanana suddenly awoke. He was off that couch in an instant and headed for the door to wake the Brazilians to take us to the hospital.

As Xanana beat on my mother's door to rouse her, it occurred to me that I hadn't felt any contractions. Didn't all the books say that the contractions began before the waters broke? I phoned Teresa, apologised for waking her and explained what had happened, and she told me to come in to the hospital so she could give me a once-over.

We left my mother scanning my pile of pregnancy books and headed for Bidau, the suburb in the eastern part of Dili where the hospital was. The Brazilians didn't look too annoyed at having been woken—they probably thought it was a false alarm as I wasn't yet writhing in pain.

Teresa was waiting at the side entrance to the hospital when we arrived. Apart from the odd security guard and pacing visitor, it was dark and deserted. She gave me a thorough check and explained that once the waters had broken there was a risk of infection and that my little boy's exit might need to be induced if things didn't start happening on their own. She told us to go home and report back to the hospital at ten o'clock the next morning.

By the time we got home, Mum was an expert on the early signs of labour and had polished off her third cup of Earl Grey tea. I soon noticed some blood mixed with the clear 'water' which had been my baby's cocoon, so I made one last call to Teresa before heading back to bed. She told me it was probably just the show coming away, which seemed to be another sign of an upset in the correct order of things. Needless to say, I didn't manage to get much sleep between 3 a.m. and 7 a.m.

In the few hours before 10 a.m., I drank copious cups of Earl Grey tea, checked and re-checked the contents of my hospital bag and the baby's little bag, and Xanana loaded the other bits and pieces we'd need to get us through the labour—a pedestal fan, pillows and an Esky packed with drinks and snacks.

The contractions had started but were still very mild and not causing me much discomfort at all. When we got to the hospital, Teresa checked their regularity and after discovering they were between 10 and 15 minutes apart suggested a walk around the hospital grounds might encourage some action. Xanana began the walk with us but was soon waylaid by patients and their visitors, all wanting to shake his hand and stop him for a chat.

Teresa and I stopped by the cafeteria for a cold drink and at midday she repeated her examination and gave me an internal check-up. She was a bit disappointed that I hadn't dilated more than a couple of centimetres and told me she would give me until about 2 p.m. before we would need to think about putting me on a drip to induce stronger contractions. She also warned me that the drip would make the contractions much more painful than they would normally be.

I sat out the next couple of hours in the air-conditioned cubicle in the maternity ward and, thankfully, the contractions started to get stronger. But I was still smiling when Sue, an Australian midwife, popped her head in the door to check on me. She thought 'real' labour must still be some time off. 'When the time comes you won't be wearing that grin,' she joked.

Now and then Teresa checked the intervals of the contractions and the baby's heart rate and recorded every change in a little logbook. Sometime after two o'clock she did another internal examination, and was satisfied that I was dilating fast enough to not need the drip. *Thank goodness*, I thought.

Soon the contractions took complete hold of my body and I spent the next few hours battling the excruciating pain. I went through most of the labour kneeling on a mattress on the floor of the air-conditioned consultation room, with my forearms resting on Xanana's knees. He was sitting on the room's only item of furniture, a vinyl-covered sofa, and he was with me throughout it all—apart from short intervals when stress and nervousness got the better of him and he escaped outside for a cigarette.

Hours passed before I finally felt the urge to push. But when I started pushing, nothing happened. I was encouraged to experiment with a variety of positions—kneeling, squatting, prone—but the baby seemed no closer to coming out, and my physical exhaustion increased with every contraction.

Through the haze of pain and weariness, I became aware of the presence of Xanana's niece Virna. She was a doctor with a daughter of her own, and had somehow found out that I was in labour. Her voice was soon part of the chorus of calls. 'Push,' I heard. 'Push harder.'

At one point someone said it was 9 p.m.—20 hours after my waters first broke. *How much longer is this going to last?* I thought, but it never occurred to me to ask for pain relief. All I was capable of registering was that the pain was acute and it couldn't possibly go on for much longer.

I was intermittently crying out, which in East Timor is something not entirely common and definitely not encouraged as a way of managing pain. But I figured it wasn't the moment for cultural sensitivity, so I continued to vocalise my pain when the urge took me.

A short time later, Teresa checked the baby's heart rate and I gathered that there was a change and she was concerned for his well-being. She recommended to Etelvina and Virna that I be put on a drip to strengthen the contractions and accelerate the birth. Virna and Etelvina wanted me to try out some different positions, but by then I was too exhausted to move and only wanted it all to be over.

Somehow I managed to signal to Teresa my agreement. After all, I had made it clear to her in the lead-up to the birth that I was happy to be guided by her. I had every faith in her experience and superior wisdom.

Shortly afterwards, I was guided into the safe room and my legs were slung uncereimoniously into the steely stirrups of the delivery bed and a drip inserted into my arm. And just then my mother, pale with worry and anxiety, briefly appeared by my side and planted a kiss on my hair, which was plastered with sweat to my forehead and cheeks.

Another hour or so passed. The contractions grew stronger and more painful thanks to the drip, and soon Etelvina and Sue had positioned themselves on either side of the bed so that I could brace myself against them. I could hear Xanana speaking to me close by my head and the midwives' exhortations to push, but I seemed incapable of any kind of meaningful interaction with anyone as I was lost in the fog-like pain which had descended around me.

When my increasingly feeble attempts to push the baby out seemed to be getting me nowhere, I started to feel like a failure and became vaguely conscious of a decision being taken by someone. Suddenly male voices were added to those of the midwives and Xanana.

Somebody whispered in my ear that a vacuum extraction was about to be performed and that a paediatrician had been summoned to carry out the procedure. Teresa started preparing the instruments to perform an episiotomy, which was now becoming an inevitability.

Tensions among the hospital staff were high, and Teresa snapped at Etelvina when she offered some advice or a comment on what Teresa was about to do. Teresa stormed out of the room, but I managed to raise my head from the bed. 'Don't leave me,' I called out.

The lower half of my body was ablaze with an assortment of pains, which now included the sting of my cut flesh, swiftly followed by the sensation of something metallic being inserted into me. The hum of voices around me rose to an excited crescendo and I felt my baby being dragged out of my body.

And then finally, at 10.50 p.m., I heard that long-awaited sound: a baby's cry. And there he was on my stomach, all pink and slippery and perfect. I looked down and saw that Alexandre wasn't covered with any of the blood and goo I had seen in photos of newly born babies. He seemed to have come out pre-washed.

He was whisked away to be given a routine check-up by

the paediatrician and for the next half an hour or so I felt so relieved that I was free from the contractions. As Etelvina set to work on my ten stitches, I told her the pain was negligible in comparison with what I had just experienced.

Outside the room I could hear the midwives excitedly congratulating my mother, and the small crowd of Xanana's family who had gathered. My mother later told me that Xanana's sister Dina and two or three of the big, brawny Brazilian guards had rushed to her side to embrace and kiss her when Alexandre's cry was finally heard. They seemed not only to have sensed her anxiety and concern, but also shared it.

Alexandre was soon returned to me and Xanana and I had our first chance to contemplate our little son. Somehow he looked too perfect and we decided that he took after his father in the nose department, given his rather prominent, squat little nose. Xanana surprised me by how confidently he cradled the little bundle in one arm while shaking hands with all the assembled well-wishers with the other.

I wanted to put Alexandre to the breast at once and was a little unsettled when the East Timorese midwife who was then tending to me suggested it was best to wait until my milk came in. I'd read extensively about the benefits of colostrum and was confident my decision was right, so I went ahead. To my delight, Alexandre attached himself immediately to the nipple I offered him and proceeded to suckle.

I would have liked nothing better than a warm shower or bath, but the facilities didn't exist and besides, it would have been an unorthodox request. It is common for East

Timorese women to refrain from washing, particularly their hair, for 30 days after giving birth.

By the time Xanana and my mother left for home and the throngs of midwives and other curious hospital staff had dispersed, it was close to two o'clock in the morning. Alexandre, swathed in muslin wraps, was laid down to sleep by my side. It felt strange to contemplate him as a separate person as opposed to the writhing, faceless little being who had shared my body for nine months. After a while, Etelvina made a makeshift bed for Alexandre in the vestibule of the safe room so that I could get some rest. We both woke to Alexandre once or twice when he stirred and I fed him, but I only managed to fall asleep again when he had been returned to my side.

It was the height of the build-up to the rainy season and the air inside the room was warm and thick, so I kept surreptitiously turning the fan's cooling air directly on me. Etelvina was disapproving—it was thought that exposing a baby to excessive air currents would allow 'wind' to get inside the baby.

I was keen to get home as soon as possible and Xanana and my mother returned to the hospital to collect me the next morning. Teresa paid regular visits to our home in the days and weeks that followed. She helped me with breast-feeding, monitored my body's recovery from the wear and tear of labour, and answered the many questions I had on a range of issues.

Advice on these and other issues was also offered by our two East Timorese housekeepers and an assortment of neighbours and well-wishers who visited our home, often carrying traditional gifts of live chickens—chicken meat is believed to promote breastmilk production—lengths of *tais* and fruit.

Our housekeepers, Anita and Alzira, were insistent that I should feed Alexandre a mixture of honey or sugar and water before my milk came in. They also looked askance every time I ate or drank anything cold, as it is the belief in East Timor that cold beverages and food inhibit milk production. And there was more advice to come: how I should dress—warmly—and also how to settle Alexandre when he woke—by immediately picking him up and rocking him back to sleep.

I was clear about what I believed in and would practise with my son, but there were moments when all the advice caused me a good deal of stress and anxiety and, in my fragile postnatal state, I would occasionally break into tears. Having my mother around to affirm my decisions and ways of doing things was a tremendous comfort, particularly since Xanana's commitments meant he was frequently away during those first days and weeks.

In many ways, Alexandre was a tiny mascot for East Timor's infant nationhood. Many of his development milestones coincided with important developments in the life of the new nation of Timor-Leste. He ate his first solids on the day the new defence force was established and had begun making 'blah, blah' noises with his tongue by the time election plans were announced for Constituent Assembly members. Alexandre's was the first birth to be registered with the new UN-established Civil Registry and he attended many of the receptions and parties that marked important events.

The birth of our second son, Kay Olok, on 11 August

2002 at Dili National Hospital, now the central health facility of the Ministry of Health of the Democratic Republic of Timor-Leste, was a relatively rapid affair. The labour only lasted about three hours and this time there was no need for intervention of any kind. I was also prepared for and more immune to the barrage of advice and comments I received in that postnatal period.

Our third son, Daniel Sword, was born at Dili National Hospital at 2.30 a.m. on 17 November 2004. Labour lasted only about one-and-a-half hours and the midwife, Etelvina, who had delivered our other two boys, saw Daniel safely into the world. Xanana was by my side throughout and my mother was also there—it was the first time in her life she'd witnessed a baby being born.

After having three children, I really do wonder how the average East Timorese woman manages to give birth to and raise 7.5 children. At the same time, having children around us keeps Xanana and me focused on the future—of our family and of our country—as we both grapple with the tremendous challenges associated with rebuilding Timor-Leste. We really have a duty to our children as much as to all East Timorese to do that job well.

Postscript

Kirsty became First Lady of one of the poorest nations in the world when her husband Xanana Gusmão was made President of the Democratic Republic of East Timor on 19 May 2002.

Shortly after giving birth to Alexandre, Kirsty was asked by UNICEF to endorse its efforts to promote exclusive breastfeeding for the first six months of life in East Timor. 'Exclusive breastfeeding is quite literally a matter of life and death in East Timor,' says Kirsty, who was born in Melbourne in 1966 and grew up in Melbourne and Bendigo. 'An alarmingly high number of children die before they reach their first birthday as a result of preventable conditions such as diarrhoea and malnutrition, often caused by the premature introduction of complementary feeding.'

It is common for East Timorese mothers to introduce supplementary foods after just three months, a situation Kirsty says is both unnecessary and dangerous, especially with the absence of a clean water supply and the difficulty of sterilising bottles.

In 2003, Kirsty set up the country's first breastfeeding body, the Klibur Susubeen Inan Nian ba Kosok Oan (Breastfeeding Association of Timor-Leste) to promote the benefits of breastfeeding. The association is under the umbrella of the Alola Foundation, an organisation she established in 2001 to promote better health for women and children in her adopted country.

Kirsty insists on travelling with her boys 'unless completely impractical', and can be seen at official functions with her children wrapped around her legs. But still, she says she finds combining motherhood and being a stateswoman the 'same challenge that it is for any working mother anywhere in the world'.

While she admits to feeling overwhelmed by the 'guilt and sense that one never manages to achieve the right balance of commitment to work and family', life has become more manageable since acquiring a personal assistant.

Meanwhile, it seems her husband, who has two children from a previous marriage, has achieved much of the joy his fortune-telling friend predicted in 1994. 'Xanana derives a great deal of pleasure from the boys. They help to keep him grounded and his sense of fun and humour alive.'

For more information about Kirsty Sword Gusmão's Alola Foundation, visit: www.alolafoundation.org.

'I had a choice and I chose a Caesarean'

SNEZNA KEREKOVIC

I met George in 1987 when I was 22 and he was 21. We both worked part time at Grace Bros in the city—he was the elevator operator, I was the information desk chick—and four years later we were married.

We never really talked about having children before we married, and afterwards it wasn't an issue. We were young and it was so far removed from our thinking. I was never the type of woman who thought, *Oh, I can't wait to have a baby, I can't wait to give birth*, and even when we reached our thirties we'd joke about the fact that neither of us was particularly clucky. We were just never that way inclined.

We cruised along happily and were very busy. I was working as an editor in trade publications, George worked for an airline and we travelled a fair bit. I told George I wasn't sure if I wanted to have kids and for a couple of years we actually contemplated a life without children.

I don't really know what changed, but when I turned 36, we started to think about it more seriously. Neither of us had a huge longing to experience parenthood but we agreed that it probably would be sad for us if we didn't have a child. I guess we were just getting older and realised we didn't really have much time to wait. But we weren't desperate—we would have waited longer if it weren't for the biological clock—and if it didn't happen naturally, we decided we wouldn't go through IVF.

It was a practical rather than emotional decision and was all very methodical. We went on one last five-week holiday to Thailand and started trying then. Four months later we were pregnant.

I'd always thought I'd have a Caesarean if I ever had a child. A lot of my friends had already had babies and they were all very keen to share their graphic stories with me. Most sounded horrific. *Oh God, I couldn't do that*, I thought. I had an absolute terror of pain and a Caesarean seemed so much more civilised.

But it really wasn't until I fell pregnant that I started seriously thinking about the process. I was surprised how much I enjoyed the pregnancy—I thought it was going to be hideous—and I actually thought it might be nice to experience a vaginal birth. It must have had something to do with those maternal surges rushing through, but I really didn't think about it all too much.

Both George and I wanted to know what sex the baby was as soon we could—we couldn't understand why you wouldn't—and at 20 weeks we found out the baby was a girl and we named her Isabella. The ultrasound also showed that my placenta was covering my cervix, so my obstetrician said I might have to have a Caesarean after all.

And that's what got me thinking. Up until six months

I'd avoided reading about birth and I actually had to tell all my friends to stop telling me their stories—I just really didn't want to know. But as time got closer I started to think about my options and did some research. I looked at the pros and cons of both a Caesar and a natural birth and read copious amounts of stuff; by then I had my own public relations business which specialised in health, so I knew exactly where to look and was on the Internet every night.

I told George I was seriously considering an elective Caesar. 'You're the one who's got to go through this,' he said. 'As long as we're not going to put you or the baby in a situation which is unsafe, then whatever you decide is fine.'

I've never had anything happen that's been really painful, but I just don't have a good tolerance to pain. Even the smallest things, such as little needles, freak me out. I'm a wuss and it doesn't take a genius to figure out that giving birth to something that's so much bigger than what it's coming out of was going to be bloody painful. It petrified me. Also, my husband's six foot four and a big, solid guy, and I'm little, so I kept thinking, *What if the child is ginormous?* And there were the after-effects as well—I knew it would never have been the same down there again.

It also seemed that every friend I had who'd recently given birth ended up having an emergency Caesar. One of them went through a horrendous 30-hour labour and afterwards was told there was no way she could have given birth naturally because her birth canal was too narrow. I really didn't want to go through hours and hours of labour and then have to have a Caesar. It would have been like a double whammy of pain and agony.

But the main attraction of a Caesarean was the control. I am a complete control freak and with a Caesarean I'd know exactly what was going to happen, when it was going to happen. You really don't know how a natural birth is going to go until you start going through it and I didn't want any surprises.

Work was an issue too. It was very important for me to know exactly when I needed to finish up. And rightly or wrongly, to me the controlled environment of an operating theatre seemed like the safest option for the baby. I was older and conscious of the health risks and I was really scared of all the things that could go wrong with natural childbirth. Sure, a Caesarean was major abdominal surgery, but it was in a controlled environment and was performed on a daily basis. In terms of a safe, healthy delivery, I reckoned there would be less stress and trauma on the child, as well as on me.

I first broached the subject with my obstetrician at my six months check-up. 'I'm just starting to think about an elective Caesarean,' I said nervously. I was expecting judgements, but he didn't make any. He just listed the advantages of both natural childbirth and a Caesarean, and he also talked about what could go wrong. I suspect that doctors probably prefer women having Caesars—they can work around their golfing days and there are no phone calls at two in the morning—but he didn't push me one way or the other. It was all coming from me.

It was quite stressful not knowing which way to go. I went through stages when I would say to myself, *Oh, for*

God's sake get over yourself. Women have given birth since the year dot. Stop being ridiculous. And then I'd think, *Oh my God, I can't do it. I don't know if I'd handle it well.* It was like I had this little devil on my shoulder talking to me. I was weighing up the options, but I was leaning towards the Caesarean even though the placenta eventually moved away from my cervix. The pros of a Caesar came to far outweigh the pros of a natural birth.

We'd booked our antenatal classes and a midwife was due to come to our house. 'Look, I'm going to be honest with you,' I told her. 'I'm 90 per cent sure that I'm going to have an elective Caesarean.' She asked me why and I told her all my concerns, but she was keen for me not to make a decision until we'd met. She thought I'd change my mind once I saw those birthing videos.

She turned up, and at the end of the lesson she said, 'Now, I'm going to put this video on.' But I didn't want to see it. 'Trust me,' I said. 'I'm not the type that would want to see this video.' I wasn't interested in graphic exposure.

'What about you, George?' she implored. 'No, not really,' he said. But she persisted and we eventually agreed. First we saw the natural birth. Someone else might have had a completely different perception of it, but all I saw was this screaming, panting, sweating woman on all fours, with an excruciating look of horror and pain on her face. It went for ages and ages and was like a barbaric, animalistic experience. George and I both sat there going, 'Right.' And then we had the lady with a Caesar. She was wheeled into the operating theatre, given an epidural, and was numb. They showed the screen over her stomach and all of a sudden the baby popped up. She was wheeled away and the baby went with the father. Then she was back in her room, holding the baby and smiling. And everything was hunky-dory.

'So, how was that?' the midwife said at the end of it. 'Well,' I replied, 'that's completely convinced me I'm having a Caesarean.' And she looked at me as if to say, 'I've got no hope with this woman.'

I think she expected me to think, *Oh my God, what an amazing experience*, whereas my reaction was, *Oh my God, what a horrendous experience that I don't want to go through, thanks very much.* People assume that every woman is going to go ga-ga over the birth experience and I just don't think that's true. Every woman is different and the decision was very black and white to me.

I went to my eight months check and a female locum was standing in for my regular obstetrician. 'I note here you're having an elective Caesar,' she said. *Here we go*, I thought, waiting for the lecture. But instead she said, 'I would never say this to anyone else, but because you've already decided to do this—I had my first child naturally and the second via a Caesar and can I tell you, I would never go natural again.' And I instantly thought, *I've made the right decision*. She was an obstetrician and a mother and she'd gone through both. There really was nothing putting me off it.

My mother had a really horrendous and dangerous birth with my younger brother—I was nine and old enough to remember—and when I told her I was going to have a Caesar she thought it sounded great. 'If I had that option open to me,' she said, 'I would have probably done the same thing.'

But not everyone was so accepting. People were a bit

incredulous and you could see some thought I was a freak. 'Don't you think it's all a bit too clinical? Don't you want to experience what it's like to give birth?' they'd ask. And I would just say, 'No, I never have. This is the way I am.' I never felt that I needed to go through the birthing process to feel more like a woman or more like a mother or attached to my child.

I felt very comfortable once I'd made the decision. I could relax and slept easily at night. My obstetrician set a date for Wednesday, 6 July 2001, a week before I was due, and I felt comforted by the fact that I knew what date I was going in, what time, how long it was going to take and when I was expected to be out. There was a sense of control over the thing, rather than fretting about when my waters would break. The only stressful thing was worrying that the baby might decide to come early, but thank goodness, she didn't.

I had planned to take a couple of months off work after the birth, so I finished on the Friday and George and I spent the weekend in a nice city hotel and luxuriated. I was really relaxed and looking forward to her arriving.

We had an early dinner the night before the operation—I wasn't allowed to eat after seven o'clock that night—and I woke up the next morning as rested as a nine months' pregnant woman could be. We drove off to the hospital and all I could think about was how we were leaving home, just the two of us, and then we'd come home as three. I was really calm. I wasn't scared about the process. The hardest part for me was always going to be the epidural. I was terrified at how painful that would be and that something could go wrong.

We arrived at the hospital at eleven, filled in my admission forms and were taken to a temporary room in the maternity ward. My obstetrician came in and talked me through what was to happen and then we had to wait until two o'clock in the afternoon.

And that was not a good time. There was nothing to do. I couldn't eat, so George and I just sat around talking and I started to get a bit nervy. Someone came in to anaesthetise my hand for a glucose drip and the thought of the epidural was really starting to freak me out, especially after I was given a brochure that explained how you could be paralysed if things went wrong. I knew once I had that I'd feel no pain, but I started to get shit scared.

Eventually, they wheeled me down to pre-op with my husband by my side. My palms were sweaty and George told me later that I looked absolutely terrified. I was white and I wasn't talking to anybody.

The anaesthetist asked me to lean over a pillow on the side of the bed and I just focused on trying not to move. I didn't want to jeopardise anything they were doing. But they had trouble getting the epidural needle in and I literally thought I was going to have a heart attack. They had to have another stab at it, but it was fine. It actually didn't hurt that much. It just felt like intense pressure had been placed on my back and within minutes I had no feeling from my waist down. They also put in a catheter.

It was weird having no feeling in my legs and I tried to lift myself onto the operating table. 'No, no,' a nurse said. 'You're not going to be able to do that. Just lie back.' They hoisted me up and by about two o'clock I entered the theatre.

It was a really gleaming, sparse, clean and clinical room and I liked that. I felt comforted by all that spareness and when I lay back all I could see was this bright light above me and George right next to me. There was also a green sheet up below my chest.

The nurses were lovely and kept the conversation light. I chatted away to George and went into a mindset that I wasn't going to think about what was happening. *They can do what they have to down there and all I care about is seeing my baby alive and well at the end of it.* I think you'd freak out if you thought about it too much.

The obstetrician and his assistant were chatting and the nurses were laughing and all this banter helped me relax. It wasn't a tense atmosphere, which made me feel confident that they knew what they were doing. Everything was under control.

George was talking to distract me so I couldn't really hear what was going on but I could smell the laser burning through my skin. I could sense a bit of pulling and tugging, and the next thing my obstetrician said, 'Get a load of this!' I couldn't see and wondered what was going on. 'What's happening?' I asked George. And he smiled: 'She's coming out with her middle finger sticking up.' I was so relieved. 'That would be right,' I said.

It all seemed so quick. She came out crying and they wrapped her up straight away and brought her to me so I could cuddle her and say hello. And that was a lovely surprise—I'd always been under the impression that she'd be whisked off after the Caesar, but she wasn't.

I'd never thought I wouldn't bond with my baby and there it was, a definite, immediate bonding. I felt this was the most amazing thing we'd ever done and probably would ever do. She came out looking so cute and wasn't squashed up at all. She was beautiful and I felt such a surge of love.

George went with the midwife to give Bella her first bath and I was sewn back up and taken down to post-op. But all I wanted to do was be back up with George and Bella. I was so impatient, but they had to check my blood pressure and keep an eye on me.

For some reason I'd assumed that you didn't bleed from your vagina when you had a Caesar, but you do, and the nurses came in and changed my pads, which was all a bit gross. They were also waiting for me to regain some feeling in my lower half.

I was there for about half an hour and when they finally took me up to the maternity ward, George and Bella weren't there. They eventually arrived and he put her on my chest. We both sat and gazed at her adoringly and I breastfed her for the first time. That first breastfeed was lovely and made me bond with her even more.

I felt absolutely fine. I wasn't tired. It just wasn't an exhausting or tiring process apart from the stress factor of having the epidural. I didn't have to do a thing. I just got wheeled in. I had the pethidine attached to my back so there was no pain—I'd press a little button whenever I felt anything—and before I went to sleep that night I had regained some feeling in my legs, which was reassuring.

The next morning I woke up really early—Bella was still in the nursery—and I could feel my legs move. I called the midwife and asked if I could have a shower. She came and took the catheter out, and I got up very easily. I had a shower—with the pethidine drip attached—blow-dried my hair and then sat up in bed and waited for my visitors.

I was incredibly mobile and was only on the drip for a couple of days before I went on to Panadeine Forte. I felt little twangs of pain near the scar, but never to the point where it was debilitating. It was pain that even I could deal with. A girlfriend who'd had a baby vaginally a year earlier visited me in hospital and was astounded. 'I couldn't walk properly for six weeks afterwards,' she said. I was swanning around.

My expectation was always that it would take a while to recover from the Caesarean and I was prepared for a lot of pain. It's major abdominal surgery—you can't kid yourself about that—but after a week I was home and able to do everything. There were no dramas lifting and bathing Bella and I took Panadol if I ever felt any pain. The scar has never bothered me—it's so low and so faint you can hardly see it. And I was back running twice a week four weeks after I had Bella.

Some women go through a lot more pain postoperatively than I did. Others think they're mentally prepared for a Caesar, then afterwards find it quite traumatic and have other complications. I didn't. I look at Bella, this very robust, happy, healthy little girl, and to me that's the main thing and it was successful. She was the perfect baby and I really don't think she will feel any grief on missing out on a vaginal birth. If anything, she'll be very pleased that she was quite the centre of attention.

You read a lot of stuff about celebrities having elective Caesars and being 'too posh to push', but that's ridiculous. Sure, if I wasn't in the financial position I was, I wouldn't have had the choice, but it had nothing to do with being too posh to push. If I didn't have the choice of an elective Caesarean, I would have given birth more conventionally and I would have dealt with it. But because of modern surgery advances and health care practices, I did have a choice and it was the right choice for me. It worked.

Postscript

While bonding with Isabella was never a problem for Snezna, breastfeeding was. 'I had the worst time with breastfeeding,' she says. 'Every time I fed it was like someone was driving a knife into my breast.'

Snezna says she had a lot of support from medical practitioners about her choice to have a Caesar, but not so with breastfeeding. 'I had a midwife come here at home a number of times when I really wasn't coping and the message was persevere,' says Snezna, who would cry in pain every time she breastfed. 'Not once did one of them suggest I stop breastfeeding and convert to a bottle.'

Snezna, who works from her inner-western, Sydney home, took two months off work, and says she was struggling to cope in those first few months. But when she gave up breastfeeding at three months, things changed. 'As soon as I stopped breastfeeding it was a completely different scenario,' she says. 'It was like a huge pressure had been lifted. The hardest thing to cope with when I was breastfeeding was just not being in control. Must be my personality.'

Snezna and George were committed to having just one child—'We were really happy with Bella and wanted to give her the best of everything'—but after seeing their daughter interact with other children have recently had second thoughts. But Snezna insists she won't have another child beyond 40. 'We're giving ourselves a year,' she says, 'and if it doesn't happen, that's it.' And the birth will be by Caesarean.

Despite Snezna's reluctance to have children in her twenties, she says she'd probably have tackled parenthood differently if she had her time again. 'Now that we've done it, I think we were mad,' she says. 'I wish I'd done it when I was twenty bloody six. It's easier when you're younger.'

A very public pregnancy

AMANDA KELLER

Harley and I had been trying to have a baby for a long time. We'd been married for more than ten years, I was in my late thirties, working on breakfast radio with Andrew Denton, and it was something we really wanted. I used to hate people telling me to relax or that I shouldn't be working so hard. Their insensitivity used to stun me. 'Oh, you don't have kids,' some would say, and it was really hurtful. You don't always choose these things.

But I never spent years sitting it out waiting for a baby. I've got friends who gave up work to try and have families and have ended up without the baby, without a job, and still haven't found a way back into the workforce. Being busy kept me going and I didn't want to get to 50 and think I'd lived a half-life. Having a baby wasn't the driving force in our lives. We were getting on with it and in the midst of that were trying to have a baby.

I probably didn't realise how much I wanted a baby, but there were times when it hit me unexpectedly. Harley is a Kiwi and in August 1999, we went on a skiing holiday to Queenstown. One night I had a dream and in it I could feel the weight of a baby in my arm. The next morning I woke up and I could still feel the warmth of the baby, and I sat with Harley in this beautiful place and just bawled.

I never assumed we would have a baby, so when I found out I was pregnant at the age of 38 I was astonished. I was thrilled and excited, but then my brain clicked in. *I know this collection of cells has to go a journey yet before it's a recognised thing to believe*, I thought. *I've got to wait twelve weeks before I can accept this.*

A year earlier my best friend Vanessa's baby died during childbirth, and in a way that skewed my view of statistics. Vanessa had gone into her pregnancy never doubting for a second that she would have a baby, and although I didn't think anything bad would happen to me, I didn't presume a pregnancy equalled a healthy, living baby.

I was cautious, but Harley was the opposite. 'Nope,' he said. 'Let's celebrate. If it doesn't go any further, we'll be sad either way but at least we're here.' He really wanted to let rip and was very different to how I expected he'd be. We almost swapped roles.

I thought I would be panicky and nervous throughout the pregnancy but I wasn't. I had a dreamy, floaty pregnancy, and after trying for all those years the world really seemed a different place. I didn't have any morning sickness and at one point early on I thought it would actually be nice to have a day of it, just so I had some physical evidence. But then I'd see friends laid low with it and think, *God, why would I ever wish for that*?

I talked a lot about the pregnancy with Andrew on air. When I look at it now, it was a real risk considering what had happened to Vanessa, but that was my whole job. We shared our lives with our listeners and they shared theirs with us so it seemed the most natural thing to say, 'Hey, I'm pregnant.'

Getting up at 4.20 a.m. for work each day actually suited me. I was waking up early anyway and I'd come home and sleep all afternoon. And it was great fun to go to work. I really enjoyed it. We didn't know whether we were having a boy or a girl so we named the baby 'Norbit' and people would always come up to me and say, 'How's the pregnancy going? How's Norbit?' but it never felt invasive.

I planned to work right up to the birth but not because I was superwoman. I had an on-air contract that only allowed three months maternity leave. I knew I had a limited time so instead of giving myself the luxury of taking a month off before the birth, I wanted to take that time with the baby. I also thought the minute I didn't feel well I'd stay at home, but I felt great—it was a wonderful, thrilling time—and it really took my mind off it all.

I never obsessed about Vanessa's experience but it was still so raw. Even when we did the hospital tour at 35 weeks and the guide said, 'When you come in to have your babies, they'll be delivered here,' I looked around the room and thought, *How naive if we all think we're going to be given living babies.* Being older made me realise that there were risks and that you don't always get a happy result.

I wasn't very big and at 36 weeks I had an ultrasound to check to see if the baby was getting the nutrients it needed. I was a small baby, and this baby wasn't massive, but after the scan the ultrasound guy called in a doctor for a chat. 'Are you booked in at the hospital?' he asked. 'No,' I said. They thought my cervix was four centimetres dilated and I was amazed. 'I am such a goddess,' I thought. 'I'm halfway through labour and I didn't even know.' But, of course, my obstetrician did an internal examination and I wasn't at all—my cervix just somehow looked that way on the scan.

I got a little bit concerned at work towards the end of my pregnancy. Triple M was a very blokey station and although I'd known Andrew for 20 years and loved him dearly, I thought if my waters broke in front of him I'd have to kill myself and the other blokes too. I once showed them my big, round, pregnant stomach and they were like, 'Er, yuk, yuk.' They would have screamed like girls if they'd witnessed anything icky.

About ten days before my late May due date, Andrew and I saw *Joe Dirt*, this terrible David Spade film. And I thought, *Can you imagine if my waters broke in this cinema, and I'd have to tell my child I was watching the worst film of all time when he was born?* They didn't, thank God, and that night I started reading a birthing book a friend had lent me. It described how to see pain as power and how your uterus would open like a flower during labour and it all sounded good.

I was really looking forward to labour. I knew I had a decent pain threshold and wasn't a wuss and I thought it would be a giant challenge. I didn't have a birth plan though. I didn't think the birth was about me. It was all about a healthy baby coming out and I didn't care how we did it. I also trusted my obstetrician, a wonderfully gentle man, to make the decisions for me.

I went to work the next day and we interviewed David Spade. We took all these photos of the three of us in mullet wigs with my stomach sticking out. I bought some fish and went home to have lunch with Harley, who works from home. I sat down at the table and suddenly my waters broke. I knew the baby might come early because of my age, but I got such a shock. I really had no inkling it was all about to happen. I was very relieved they'd broken at home and was just so excited. I phoned the hospital and the midwife told me to put some frozen peas on my stomach to check to see if the baby moved and I did that and felt the baby jumping around.

I had read enough to know that it could be days before I'd need to go into the hospital, but then some period-like pain started. 'Oh, okay,' I said. 'This is all right.' Then all of a sudden it went from mild, extremely manageable pain to full-on, unbelievable agony. I'd never had pain like it and I was completely knocked sideways by it. I couldn't brace against it or work with it or fight it in any way. I found it extraordinary. Straight away it was like I was in the surf and being drowned, and I could not believe that for generations women had gone through this and hadn't told me. But how could you tell someone? How could you prepare for it? And when I look back at it, God, how stupid that I was actually looking forward to it.

The hospital told us to come straight in and the drive was excruciating. I sat there strapped in with these waves in my stomach turning me inside out and I couldn't do anything but try to make a noise to get through it. We got to the hospital in about five minutes and I climbed out of the car and the next thing I knew I was on all fours, roaring, in the carpark.

Eventually, I made it up to the delivery suite, and I was trying to recall the mantra 'Pain equals power and my uterus is opening like a flower'. Instead my mantra was 'I can't do this. I can't do this. Frig the flower'. My midwife checked my cervix and I was four centimetres dilated. *Imagine getting here and not knowing?* I thought, remembering that earlier ultrasound.

You just never know how you are going to be in labour and I was strangely polite. I didn't yell or scream and at one stage I even asked Harley, 'May I please have a glass of water?' I may have been polite but I knew what I wanted. The midwife said, 'How about I just run you a hot bath?' And I said, 'How about you inject me in the back with a needle?' She asked again, but I gave the same response so they called up the anaesthetist.

I'm sure everyone falls in love with her anaesthetist. I had the shakes badly after the epidural, but I didn't care because I was out of pain. I looked on that machine and could see there was a contraction but couldn't feel a thing and that just felt fantastic.

I watched a bit of television and snoozed and I think I must have been a bit out of it because they brought in a meal for Harley and told me not to eat it. But I ate the whole thing—tomato soup, sandwiches, everything—and then threw it all back up again for about an hour. That third stage of labour apparently makes you nauseous and with all that food, I just vomited for ages.

By about ten o'clock that night, it came time to push and even though they'd turned down the epidural, I couldn't feel a thing. I was making the face of pushing and hoping I was—the next day my face and shoulders ached—but I really had no way of knowing if it was helping.

The baby was taking a long time to come out—he just wasn't budging—and in the end my obstetrician got the vacuum thing and at 11.30 p.m. on 22 May 2001, he pulled him out. Harley and I had seen videos of misshaped heads in our antenatal classes, and we'd laughed and laughed, and out came Liam looking like Nefertiti. He was this scrawny, skinny thing in a space blanket with this strangely shaped head that they'd covered with a little knitted cap straight away. I had to press down on the cap to make sure it wasn't all head.

They gave him to me to hold and there was no instant, 'Isn't he gorgeous?' He was like a newborn cat and almost reminded me of Shrek with these animatronic eyes opening to look at me. It was still quite mind-blowing. *We're going to be looking at each other, hopefully for the rest of my life*, I thought, but I didn't have an instant rush of love. It wasn't that I didn't love him. I was just so overwhelmed by the trauma of labour. I was in shock and didn't feel much more after that.

Liam had been crossing his legs in the womb. 'I'll just pull them down a little bit,' the doctor said and I thought, *Oh no, his legs will be malformed for the rest of his life*. I realise now that a lot of babies do that in the womb but I had no perspective that this was just normal stuff. Instead of thinking what a perfectly formed, gorgeous thing he was, I just thought, *Oh God, what's wrong?* Reality really crashed the minute he was born.

I was supposed to go to work the next morning, so by midnight Andrew and my producer knew that Liam had been born and the next morning I went on air from the hospital to break the news. Andrew was concerned about the baby and it seemed perfectly natural to share the whole experience with him and the listeners. A nurse came in to check my stitches as I spoke on air. 'Excuse me,' I whispered. 'I'm just on the phone.'

I'm surprised at how lucid I was, given I was so emotional. I was in tears, Andrew was in tears and listeners called up and they were in tears. They played a song for us—'Arms Wide Open', by Creed—and both Harley and I started bawling.

I think they were lucky they got me then because I was pretty much out of it for the rest of the week. I don't know if it had anything to do with Vanessa's experience, but I continued to feel that things weren't the way they should be and I found it just so traumatic. Liam was jaundiced and he wouldn't feed because he was so small—only 2.4 kilos—so he was in special care. He was just tired and wasn't waking up, so in the end he had to be fed by a tube.

I didn't get any of the euphoria of a new baby. I was in tears a lot of the time and I'm not normally a teary person. My nephew had a liver transplant when he was two and a lot of that started with jaundice and I'd see my baby on a table with this light on him and I'd just be bawling inappropriately.

The nurses tried to say, 'It's all right, it's all right', but I didn't want to be touched. I felt slightly embarrassed because I was aware I was over-reacting—I'd had a healthy baby and a normal delivery and for many families it was so much worse—but by then I wasn't in control of my emotions at all. He seemed so fragile and even though he'd just had a couple of little complications, I couldn't get a grip. I felt totally out of control and was on this ride just trying to hold on. I could control everything while he was inside me but now it was completely out of my hands and it was terrifying.

I was in hospital for nine days and all the flowers had bloomed and died and my room smelt. I had to have a catheter in because I'd got an infection when the vacuum pull scraped my bladder, and no one told me how much it hurt when your milk comes in—there were these big plates in my breasts—and I also had stitches. My room was dark and although I'm not prone to depression I started to get anxious. 'Can we move her to a room where there's light?' Harley asked the midwives.

That week was horrible. On the day we left the hospital, I saw a pregnant woman going in to give birth and I was almost jealous of her. I was so nostalgic for my pregnancy—that was the bit I loved—and she had all of that ahead of her whereas I just had to get on with the hard work of it.

I felt the circus had really moved on from me when we first brought Liam home. Harley was tending to the baby and I sat there and felt the most physically miserable I had ever felt in my whole life. I didn't need any help when people used to ask me how I was going during the pregnancy, but now I was suffering, everyone had moved on.

Liam still wasn't feeding so I had a lactation consultant come to my home. If a stranger knocked on your door and said, 'Let's play with your nipples', you'd probably have them arrested. But there was I saying, 'Come on in. Do what you will. Get this baby eating.'

I really didn't feel myself for a long time after Liam was born, but by the time I was due back at work in September he had put on weight and it had pretty much all come together. I didn't have much time off but in a way it was good to have a date to go back. If it had been open-ended it would have been a really tough decision because I don't think you ever feel completely ready to go back.

I thought I'd take it easy those first days and leave straight after the show but it was the week of the September 11 tragedy. That day we were on air for six hours instead of three. I hadn't had to concentrate for so long and there were kids on the phone in tears and I had this baby at home. *What's happening in the world?* I thought. My breasts were about to hit the opposite wall and at one point I started to see spots, so it was a really hard week to be back at work. But eventually things settled down and with the help of our wonderful nanny, working the early hours again suited us well.

Harley and I started to think about having another child when Liam was a year old. I wanted a sibling for Liam although I wasn't desperate for another baby, and after last time I thought it might never happen. But with my body up and running and raring to go, I fell pregnant really quickly.

This time I was relaxed enough to realise that as soon as I was past the 12-week mark, I was having a baby. I accepted I could have a healthy baby as I'd already done it and there wasn't that thing in my mind that it all wouldn't necessarily end well.

Andrew had finished at Triple M and I was now working with Mikey Robbins and Peter Berner. On Friday, 16 May 2003, when I was nearly 38 weeks pregnant, we had a blokey baby shower. We showed football games on the wall and listeners came in and gave me things like stubby-holders for the baby.

The night before I'd gone into labour with Liam, our dog Ripley had acted really strangely. She tried to get up on my lap and was very sooky and clinging, and we realised later that she must have detected the hormones shifting in the pack. So this time around, we were monitoring her very closely. Whenever she came near me, we'd be like, 'Oh my God, oh my God.'

We went out for dinner on that Saturday night with some friends. I felt uncomfortable all night and the next morning, I felt dreadful. 'Oh, it's the rich food,' Harley said.

I was lying on the couch feeling dodgy and Liam, who was nearly two and needed to be watched, was running around madly. Harley was on the phone to New Zealand all morning—his parents were buying a house and he was their power of attorney—so I couldn't go back to bed.

I had a bit of a show around lunchtime and although there were no signals from Ripley at all, I suddenly realised that life was about to change. I knew that a sibling was going to be the best thing in the world for Liam, but he was still such a baby. I looked at him and thought, *You poor bugger*, and started sobbing.

I'd been timing things when I'd been feeling yuk in the morning but there was no pattern. Still, I said to Harley, 'This might be it,' and after telling the lawyer, 'My wife's having a baby. No, she's having a baby', he eventually got off the phone.

I wasn't excited this time around. I'd forgotten what labour felt like but I knew there was nothing to be excited about. Bev, our nanny, was away and so was our back-up, so Harley called some friends and asked if they could take Liam for the night. He packed Liam up and drove him there and in the 20 minutes it took I went into full-on labour, but I was still unsure if it was. There weren't waves of it—this was just constant agony.

'Quick, we've got to go to the hospital now,' I told Harley when he returned, and the ride up there was horrendous once again—I still can't go up that road without the memory of it. All I kept thinking was, *When you get there, there will be drugs. When you get there, there will be drugs.* And as soon as I got there, at 2 p.m., I was on all fours in the carpark again.

I was clinging to the walls as we made our way up to the maternity ward and a woman came past and spoke to me. 'Amanda, you're in for your second,' she said calmly. 'I've just had my fourth.' I tried to pull my face into the approximation of a smile, but I think it came out as a roar, and when I got to the delivery suite I couldn't sit down. I was in agony and the midwife checked my cervix. 'You're fully dilated,' she said. And I was overwhelmed with the horror of knowing what that meant. I couldn't have drugs.

'Are you feeling the urge to push?' she asked. I hadn't felt it last time, so I just didn't know what to expect. 'No,' I said. 'Well, you will soon,' she said. *Thank God*, I thought, *The baby's about to be born. This pain will stop.* And then

I remembered—*Hang on, there's this whole other stage to do, that I know nothing about,* and that was frightening.

I stayed on that bed in a ball and tried to use the gas. I had no success with it during Liam's birth but this time I was better at it and psychologically it gave me something to do. And I was very polite again. 'Oh dear, oh dear,' I kept saying. 'Excuse my language,' I said to the doctor at one point. He didn't realise I was joking. 'Oh, we see a lot worse than that,' he said, and I'm quite capable of a lot worse than that. I'm a good swearer but I was being so polite, even to Harley, who wouldn't have minded if I were cranky.

I didn't want any talking. I didn't want any soothing or massaging. It was like I had a bell over my head and I was just bunkered down and getting through it.

I'd asked Harley before I went into labour to tell me that all this pain meant we were getting closer, but as soon as he said that I said, 'Oh, shut up.' All the things I told him to say were suddenly irritating, so I said 'Shut up' quite a few times.

Just before five o'clock, I felt this fizzing in my bum as if I had to do a giant poo and I suddenly said 'Oooooooo.' 'That's it,' said my midwife. 'That's the urge to push.'

I imagined I would give birth doing a big squat but I was lying on my side with my leg up and I had to push, push, push. It was just like in the movies—'One more, one more,' they all said—and there was this rush and a hot whoosh, which was a very nice feeling, and then voompa, out Jack came.

He was still a small baby, but he was much fleshier than Liam was, and I knew what newborns looked like so there wasn't that shock. He was given an absolutely clean bill of health, and when he started feeding straight away I felt as in control as I could possibly be. *Okay*, I thought. *I know this.*

Either I was different or he was just perfect but I knew the stuff that didn't matter and it was a very different story from that first time. I had a very restful night and the next morning I opened up the curtains in the hospital room—I had a light one this time—and I said out loud through the window, 'There is a new person in the world and his name's Jack.'

It was never my intention to have a drug-free birth—I was thinking about drugs from Jack's conception—but it was such a different post-birth experience for me. I had the euphoria and although I got a haemorrhoid and had stitches, I recovered quickly and Jack thrived. And I did feel a sense of achievement. I'd faced that pain and got through it, but birth is a huge deal no matter how you do it.

It was so busy at home that it was almost restful in the hospital and I did panic about going home. I'd left a baby there, but when Liam came in to visit he looked about eight or nine, although behaviourally he wasn't. He'd grown up overnight and part of me grieved that I'd lost my baby boy. I was also very concerned before Jack was born about how I could possibly love another baby and if I did, would that mean I loved Liam less? I thought it was a lose-lose situation. I beat myself up about that stuff but, of course, as every mother says, there's enough love to go around.

I sat at home with sore boobs, stitches and a haemorrhoid feeling miserable one night. But because it was the second time around, I knew that it was all temporary. I knew I had to take a deep breath and just put up with it.

It was bloody hard for those first few months, though. Liam got a baby for his second birthday—Jack was born four days before—and that coincided with the 'terrible twos'. I had a nanny, and Harley was at home quite a bit as well, and even so I felt like I was drowning. I don't know how mums do it on their own.

Sometimes I get a shock when I'm driving and see two baby-seats in the back of our car. I often have a euphoric burst and I get a bit teary, and other times I think, *God, how did that happen?* Harley's 53 and I'm 42 and here are two babies, and it shocks me in so many different ways. When I was a teenager I thought that at 40 you were a grandmother, and I wouldn't have believed anyone if they'd said I would have a baby at 41. But I really wouldn't have had it any other way. I know the joy of feeling the weight of a warm baby in my arms and I have a sense that we're now complete.

Postscript

Not long after giving birth to Jack, Amanda Keller left Triple M to present *Mondo Thingo* on ABC-TV and has since moved back to breakfast radio at Sydney's WS FM.

While she says she has reclaimed her pre-baby body to a 'certain extent', Amanda reckons some things may never be the same. 'I notice the breasts, I have to say,' she remarks. 'I never had big ones before but at least they were firm. After the first baby it was a bit of a tragedy, but this time, there's just no meat left.'

Amanda says that having known her producer/director husband Harley Oliver for such a long time before having children meant the couple, who live with their boys in Sydney's eastern suburbs, 'knew who we were and who we'd be at the other side of having children'. However, delayed parenthood has other more practical complications. 'If we want our boys to go to private schools, that's ten years away,' she says. 'That's the biggest expense in your lives besides your house and I'll be pension age then. The school will have to have ramps so I can drop them off and come in.'

Amanda has no regrets that she shared one of her most private experiences with a large part of Sydney and says that people still tell her they cried the day Liam was born. 'I feel really touched by that,' she says. 'I take it as such a compliment. People felt that their friend was having a baby and it was just such a lovely thing to share.'

Her unforgettable on-air moment is now on rotation on Amanda's iPod. 'It came up the other day when I went for a walk,' she says. 'I hadn't heard it for a while, and there I was, walking along the street bawling like a madwoman.' But that's not the only memory from Liam's birth that causes a reaction. 'Harley took some beautiful photos of Liam looking like Igor,' she says. 'We laugh at them now the same way we laughed at those babies on the video. We got us a beauty.'

'Mummy's tummy's broken'

ALISON BAKER

I was told I couldn't have children when I was 14. It was the early eighties, in England, and after finding a twist at the top of my uterus, the doctors said, 'That's it, forget about it, go and do something else with your life.'

It was a weird kind of discovery. I think my mother (who passed away when I was 19) was devastated whereas I was more interested in what I was going to wear to the junior disco. In a way, I guess I was lucky. I cannot imagine what it would have done to me if I'd found out at 35 after trying to fall pregnant for years. It would have been heartbreaking.

I never really thought about it during my twenties. I was busy working hard as a sales director in Sydney, making lots of money. Things changed when I met David. It was instant attraction but I was involved in another relationship. David is a very honest person so he kept his distance, but when I was single again we all started going out as a big group, and one night in an Oxford Street bar at three o'clock in the morning he uttered the immortal words, 'I fancy you.' And that was it.

It was a lovely old-fashioned courtship and I knew straight away that I wanted to have a family with this man. I felt so connected with him. We literally talked about it on the first date, so he knew right from the start that I couldn't bear children. It was all very clear from the beginning.

We seriously started thinking about having children when David asked me to marry him. I was 29 and suddenly this path was laid out for us. We knew when the wedding was going to be, and we knew we wanted a family but it was like, 'How are we going to make this happen?'

I always wanted children and had this belief I would, but hadn't quite worked out how. David very much wanted children too and he was the kind of person who made me believe everything was going to be all right. His attitude was, 'Okay. What's the plan? How can we fix it?'

We started to go through the options. IVF was out—the specialists thought I wouldn't take a child to full term, and pregnancy could be really dangerous for me as I'd had a heart operation when I was 22. A few did suggest adoption, but first and foremost we wanted to try for our own child.

We hadn't really heard of surrogacy—I don't think many people had in the early nineties—until a friend of ours who worked at the ABC rang and said she'd come across something about it. David and I decided to start researching it that night and it was a very emotional evening. I'd been very good at putting the whole issue of exactly how we would have children on the backburner and suddenly it was at the forefront of our lives.

Soon we'd done enough research to realise surrogacy might be feasible for us. We discussed it with both our families and got nothing but unequivocal support. We were bracing ourselves for negative reactions. The first group of friends we told said, 'Okay, you know a lot of people are going to think this is wrong and find it hard to support you. But we will.' I remember that horrified me. To me, surrogacy was just a normal step, admittedly a big one, from IVF. It's just assisted reproduction.

We went to a gynaecologist who was right at the top of his profession here in Sydney, and when I asked him about surrogacy he literally escorted me from his office, saying, 'It's illegal in this country, I'm not prepared to talk about it.' He was horrible. There was no sense of sympathy or support.

Commercial surrogacy is illegal in Australia. However, altruistic surrogacy, at that point, was legal in the ACT. My sister and I talked a bit about her being the surrogate, but it wasn't right for her then as she'd just had two children, and it didn't feel right for us either. And much of that probably had to do with sibling rivalry. But there were all sorts of issues. If my sister carried our child, her name would be on the baby's birth certificate with my husband's—which could just be a little too close for comfort.

We soon found Doctor Sue Craig, who runs the Artarmon practice Gynae Care. Sue was just wonderful. When we walked in, it almost felt like she was a natural healer. She was very open and told us she was working with a couple who were trying to do the same thing as us.

She passed on our details to these people, who rang to invite us to a support group meeting. So off we tootled one Sunday afternoon. It was full of people a lot older and sadder than we were. There were women who told stories of stillbirths and miscarriages and it was very emotional. The other couple had received a tape from an American company called The Center for Surrogate Parenting in California, which they showed, and we all took down the details.

We rang the company and discovered they were actually coming out to do a seminar at Darling Harbour, which we of course went to. We really liked the people. They were professional and very organised and explained all the legalities and costs involved. Some of the families they'd already worked with in Australia came and talked to us about their experiences and had lunch with us, which was lovely and very encouraging.

At that time, California was the only state in America that allowed commercial surrogacy. It also had a law that meant if a child was genetically yours, it was legally yours, and you didn't have to adopt it. You had to adopt your own child in every other place in the world.

After a couple of conversations with the head of the company and the doctor we'd be working with, we felt really confident and took them on, which involved a lot of paperwork and a lot of money.

All up it cost us about $100 000, including travel. We had to pay about $20 000 as a down payment, which went into a trust and was divided amongst the various parties once a certain level of success has been reached. There would then be more payments on the confirmation of pregnancy (around $10 000), at six months (another $10 000), then at birth ($20 000).

While people criticise surrogacy for being commercial, the system serves a very strong purpose. It's a business arrangement and is protected legally and financially for both parties. That made it possible for us to put it in a box rather than let it become overwhelming and over-emotional. And that suited us really well.

After we sent the payment over, we wrote out our story and sent some photographs, because the first thing they wanted to do was match you. And they match you very much on your and the surrogate's values and preferences, such as marital status and age, because really, it doesn't matter what religion or race you or the surrogate are.

I didn't have any preferences. I thought if another woman was prepared to do this for me, to go through six weeks of drugs, have our embryo transferred to her, a pregnancy, a delivery, and all for around $30 000, then I just didn't care. These women are not doing it for the money. They're doing it for the love and the desire. And I also trusted the agency. Their screening process was extensive.

The company sent us photos and details of a couple named Mary and Christopher, and we shared stories. I loved the look of Mary straight away and we decided to work with them. We all got tested for every kind of communicable disease, including AIDS, and then we went over to the US and spent a week with them and their two kids in Sacramento. They were just lovely.

When we got back home, the process began. I worked with my US doctor by phone. He sent a prescription to a local chemist, and then I started my meds, which was just like an IVF cycle—you take Lupron to stop ovulating and then a stimulant to produce more eggs. It's really tricky because you have to time it all so you and the surrogate mother ovulate at the same time. You can't ovulate until you're over there—you don't want your eggs to all pop out on the plane—and I was convinced I was doing the wrong thing on the wrong date.

We flew over in November, about a year after we first found the company, and I had to have a deep muscle injection mid-flight to boost my egg count. David and I went to the toilet together with a syringe. Very embarrassing.

Five days after we got there, I ovulated and had the eggs removed under a general. When I woke up, David was by my side and he'd managed to get to the shops and buy me some beautiful perfume, a card and flowers.

David had done his bit while I was under and then three days later we did a live embryo transfer to Mary. We were both there with her and we were all quite relaxed during the whole thing.

Throughout the entire process there were very clear rules about what was expected of your behaviour. And that was good. I spoke with my counsellor once a week and she'd say, 'This might be appropriate, that might not be appropriate.' So there was lots of support, which meant nobody was unsure or anxious about what they were doing.

My gut feeling about everything that went into creating this baby was, 'Yes, yes, yes,' and I was pretty much encouraged from the word go. I was 31 and when they took my eggs, they were bloody good eggs. I felt like a clucky hen and it was nice to have my body doing something right.

Then we came back to Sydney. It was around Christmas. David's parents were with us and we'd just been to see *Titanic* when we got a call from Mary saying that the transfer hadn't been successful. I was devastated. In a way it was like having a miscarriage, I'm sure not as traumatic, but we really were mentally preparing for this baby.

The reason the embryos didn't develop successfully—we'd transferred two—was that Mary had a problem with the lining of her uterus. It wasn't life-threatening and wouldn't restrict her from having more children but meant it was going to be harder for her to get pregnant.

So we were advised not to work with her any longer, and that was really hard because we'd become very close. It was particularly difficult for her because she was a first-time surrogate and was trying very hard to give this gift and it didn't work out.

But we had five frozen embryos left and the company then matched us with another couple, Kerri and Mark. Three months later, I was lucky enough to be flying to New York for work, so I flew via LA and met Kerri and Mark and their daughter, who live near LA.

I was so touched by how much trouble Kerri went to for me. I went to church with her on the Sunday and the whole congregation was fascinated by me, this woman from Australia, that 'we' were going to help. I was mobbed by people forcing knitted goods upon me. It was lovely, although somewhat overwhelming.

Surrogacy had been all new to Mary, whereas Kerri had been a surrogate mother three times before. She was a professional. This was her job. I remember Kerri once saying to me that being a surrogate mother was the only way she was going to make her mark on the world. She loved to be pregnant, she was good at it and she knew it would make an enormous difference in people's lives. And practically, it meant she could be at home with her child while making a bit of money for her family.

So I flew home and Kerri had a transfer without us a couple of weeks later. And about eight days later we got the call. It was quite early in the morning, I was in bed with David, and Kerri said, 'You're going to be a mummy.' And I wept. I absolutely wept.

It was fantastic. We kept everything crossed for the first three months and didn't tell anyone. We'd told everyone the first time around, and we just didn't want to take the risk.

I soon went to LA, again for work, and saw Kerri pregnant and it felt incredibly natural. I put my hands on her tummy and gave her a tape of us talking, which she played every night. David hadn't met her at that point and I was concerned I'd be very jealous of him touching her tummy. But when they did meet, it was all very easy and comfortable.

We were very short of money after getting together that $100 000. We didn't have our own home—we were staying at our wonderful friend Michael's place—and the three of us had this lovely winter together waiting for our little baby.

The counsellor advised us to speak with our surrogate once a week and it was our Saturday morning ritual, Kerri's Friday night. We would sit on the couch at Michael's house and talk. And those conversations never felt forced because Kerri had become a friend.

We'd talk about everything. You really do have some weird conversations, and often the blackest, darkest things are the funniest. We would scream with laughter and get ourselves in all sorts of pickles. Once we talked about what the baby might look like and I started chatting away blithely about how all David's family had big heads. 'Maybe we should stop talking about big heads,' Kerri said. 'I'm feeling kind of faint.'

We were never concerned about how Kerri was caring for the baby. I trusted her because she had been pregnant before. I hadn't. She loved her fast food, but she was always delivering incredibly healthy babies and I had enormous faith in everything she was doing.

She wanted to know the sex and we didn't, so we said, 'Fine, you go ahead, but just don't tell us.' We really felt she was a partner in the whole process and was certainly entitled to a lot of rights.

And then at about week 20, Kerri had a scan which showed a slight fault in the top of the baby's spine—potential spina bifida. She had to go for a more conclusive test and she couldn't get in for four days.

We felt completely out of control. We didn't sleep the night we waited for the results—England was playing Argentina in the World Cup—and at three o'clock in the morning the phone rang. 'It's fine, it's fine,' she said. 'Can I tell you the sex?'

And we said, 'Yes!' We wanted to know everything. We wanted to know what colour his eyelashes were. That was one of the happiest days of my life.

Then, at about 29 weeks, Kerri unexpectedly went into labour. She called and said, 'I'm in hospital, I've had some contractions.' But they gave her some drugs, she was on bed rest for a week, and they stopped. I was nearly on the plane. I was frantic. All I wanted to do was go. And this happened three times in the last ten weeks of the pregnancy.

The counsellor was just wonderful. 'Let's just think of the worst possible scenario,' she said. 'Kerri goes into labour, they can't stop it, the baby comes, you get on the plane, you're 14 hours away. I give you my word, as that baby comes, I will pick him up and I will sit and nurse him for you and I will not leave his side. You know your son will be with me. He will be protected.'

I didn't want to put the pressure of doing it all by herself on Kerri. I just didn't want to. And it wasn't something that I necessarily wanted Kerri to do either. So I thought, *That's okay. That's the worst possible scenario. We can live with that.*

But it was so hard. We didn't know whether to stay or go. I had planned to go on maternity leave three weeks before his due date and fly over two and a half weeks later, but in the end I flew out the day I left work, completely exhausted.

I'm a great one for plans and this was not going according to plan. I also wanted David to be there. I really didn't know if I could do it on my own. He was the one who took my hand and marched us down this journey. He was just completely rock solid.

I flew over a week before David and the baby didn't come, of course. So I went to the cinema, saw Kerri and Mark, had lots of dinners and then David arrived.

Kerri has had so many deliveries she knew exactly what she wanted. And being in America you can say exactly what you want. She decided to be induced at 38 weeks, on 27 November 1998, the day after Thanksgiving, so she could have a dinner for us. That also gave her time to do her Christmas shopping and give us a christening party before we left. She's very practical.

So it was quite surreal that on Thanksgiving Kerri was cooking this massive dinner for 20, and we all knew that at six o'clock the next morning we were going to be in hospital, having this baby.

It was also very exciting—we were all a bit giddy—but I was so anxious. I had to walk around the block pretending I was having breathers, but I was chainsmoking the whole time. David was really relaxed. I suppose we were like any mother and father ready to meet their baby.

The next morning we all went into the hospital together—Kerri, Mark, David and me. It was very modern and very high tech—no birthing suites or anything like that—and it was all very open. There are quite a lot of surrogates in that part of the world so our situation wasn't unusual.

Kerri had given clear directions about where she wanted us to stand for the birth—David and me on either side of her, at shoulder level, and it was all done with smoke and mirrors. She was very modest and she was in bed at all times. In the US, you don't walk around.

A bit after six o'clock she was induced with a drip and we waited. There were lots of jokes. Mark had the video set up. We painted Kerri's toenails. We had the TV on. It was as if we were waiting for the bus, and the whole time I felt a bit like the bride—kind of gracious, with very little to do. All I had to do was smile and look pretty. I felt completely useless.

An hour and a half later the contractions started quite strongly and Kerri asked for an epidural. She's tough and very knowledgeable about her body and knew when to have it. Mark and David went off to get some breakfast, and I held her while she had the epidural. She was so brave. She didn't even wince, but at that point I started to get a bit shaky. I'd always thought about meeting my baby, but at the top of my awareness was how appropriate I was with Kerri, how loving I could be to her, and I was terribly anxious about it all.

Once the epidural was in, my adrenalin started coming up. Kerri was really comfortable and we were laying bets on when the baby would arrive. The doctors' shifts changed and the new one looked like George Clooney.

She was all strapped up to a monitor so we could see the contractions and they started coming quite strongly, but then they kind of lulled off. Kerri had thought the baby would be born by ten or eleven o'clock and it got to 12.30 p.m. and there was pretty much no activity. The doctor kept coming in and then the baby's heart rate started to drop.

That was when the motherly thing kicked in. I suddenly thought, *What can I do? I'm totally out of control, I can't protect him.* The doctor told David and me to go and get a coffee—I wasn't saying anything, but I think my body language made it clear I was starting to lose it.

We went downstairs for about half an hour. When we walked back into the room, there was a very different atmosphere. It was 'game on', and the baby's heart rate had dropped right down. They were getting ready to take some pretty dramatic action.

Kerri said, 'Come and stand next to me,' and that was a big mistake. David went and stood on the other side, because those were the positions we'd agreed to, but what I hadn't realised was that I would physically need him by my side.

So I thought, *Okay, all you need to do is focus on Kerri*. I was desperate for her not to have to go through this. I loved her as a friend but I also felt responsible for the whole thing and I hadn't processed all that. And it's not like I wanted to swap places. I'm eternally grateful. But I wanted a sense of control. I'm sure a lot of fathers feel like that watching someone they love, in pain and not being able to help.

But Kerri was very reassuring. She was still not demonstrating any sense of discomfort. She just looked at me and very clearly said, 'Everything is absolutely fine.' She could have been in a supermarket queue for the amount of tension or fear she showed. She was working, she had an aim and she was not going to fail.

Kerri was listening carefully to the doctor and doing exactly what she was told. Then we had one of those awful *ER* moments where it goes from two to 14 people. 'You're not fully dilated,' the doctor said, 'but we're going to have to take the baby out.'

His heart rate was right down. 'You need to push now,' the doctor said, and Kerri held my hand and she pushed. She honestly nearly broke my heart, she pushed so hard.

I was terrified and became convinced that we'd lose him. And I didn't feel like I could do any better. I had my whole faith in Kerri, but I was utterly convinced that I wouldn't have my baby any more. I wanted to be held.

I wanted to be next to David. I wanted to run away. I didn't want to know anything about it.

I kept talking to Kerri and I was trying to come out with really sensible sentences and I wasn't listening to what the doctor said. He was saying, 'Push, push, push, stop,' and then he said, 'We're nearly there.' He got a suction cap on top of the baby's head and started to pull. I didn't hear him say, 'Stop pushing,' and I said to Kerri, 'Come on, one more big push,' and he yelled, 'No! Stop pushing now!' The baby's shoulder was stuck and the cord was around his neck.

All I could think was, *It's all over. It's all over. What a terrible waste of what we've done.* I was instantly talking myself into the fact that this baby wasn't coming and I wasn't going to be a mum. I'd never in my life done that before.

There was one more big push. And there he was, this monster. This enormous, ugly, pink, healthy, screaming bruiser.

They whizzed him off to another area of the room and to be honest, all I wanted was to be with Kerri. I kind of knew the baby, who we named James, was all right—that was starting to settle in me—and I just wanted to say thank you to her.

And Kerri sat up in bed, absolutely fine. 'Oh my God, my God,' I said to her in my high drama. 'I think that was about eight minutes of pain,' she said. 'That's not bad.' She was really chirpy and bossing people around immediately.

Throughout the whole surrogacy process the horror of birth hadn't been part of my awareness. I had no idea just how painful and violent and surreal a birthing experience really was. And I'd always considered myself to be quite good at medical things.

David cut James's umbilical cord and I went over to have a look at him and they asked me to hold this oxygen tube under his nose. I held that, in a really wobbly way, and he was just so big—nine pounds. I had had visions of a delicate little creature, but no.

Then Kerri asked for him as that was the birth plan we'd organised: the nurse would take James to Kerri and she would hand him to me because that was very much the process of saying, 'That's my part done, here's your baby.' And she did that and it was lovely.

I loved him instantly. I actually think I loved my baby from the moment we decided to make one. It wasn't like accidentally falling pregnant. It was like setting out for a gold medal where you know you're pretty determined that you're going to value it before you get there.

And it all went very quiet and peaceful. I sat with James in a chair and we just looked at him. We had half an hour of all of us, James, Kerri, Mark, David and me in the room, and then I took James to the nursery. Kerri had some stitches as she had a bad bleed afterwards, and when we came back she wanted champagne and her mum brought in sandwiches, quiche and cake for 400.

A lovely Irish nurse found us a room next to Kerri's. David and I curled up in the bed and James slept at the bottom of our bed in his crib and we kept popping around to see if Kerri was okay.

The next morning Kerri went home and we went to a nearby motel. So there we were in a motel with a 24-hour-old baby. For the first two or three days, I was an emotional wreck. I felt this weight of responsibility and terror and an overwhelming sense of, 'What do I do with this thing?' There was no midwife support, I had no family, no one was visiting me, and I wasn't in my home. I felt very disorientated. But I wasn't sore and tired, and I also wasn't breastfeeding, so I was sharing the whole experience with David from the word go.

We made all the traditional mistakes. We had the heating up so high we were in singlets, but James had a balaclava on. He was vomiting a lot, too. In Australia, you might be told by a midwife that he'd had a difficult delivery and possibly swallowed a lot of fluid and not to worry about it but, of course, in a motel at midnight in California you worry about these things. But we had Robin Barker's *Baby Love*, and we read that ferociously.

Then David had to start the tricky process of getting a birth certificate and passport. The American embassy was really good—it was used to unusual situations—but the Australian embassy was awful. I think they thought David was stealing this child. We're both on James's birth certificate. We so wanted a baby and we'd have compromised in any way possible, but ultimately those things are important and it's nice not to have had to adopt a child that's genetically ours.

Since then, we've seen Kerri twice—she and her family came over here for a holiday about two years ago, and we've stayed with them in LA and gone to Disneyland together. We speak once a month and email once a week. Some relationships with surrogates fall down, but if you're going to be friends, you're going to be friends and I think it's nice for James, too.

We made an early decision to make the birth part of our story, not a big surprise at James's sixteenth birthday. When he was about two we made him a little book, which explains how Mummy's tummy's broken and how we had to ask Kerri to help us. It's one of his favourite books.

If you asked James about it when he's older, I guess he might feel a bit of grief from missing out on that process, but being a boy I'm not sure he would. He'll probably say, 'Yeah, whatever.' He also won't have a conscious memory of the whole thing and I'm the one who is going to be grieving more than he is.

I would have loved to have carried James. I don't know how someone who has had a more traditional pregnancy feels, but I can't imagine feeling any more love, affection, worry or any of the things that parents feel towards James. I have an incredibly strong bond with him, probably too strong, but I guess I do still wish that was something I could have experienced.

And the thing I miss more than anything is the love that David would have felt towards me. I've always wanted that feeling of, 'Let my wife sit down, she's pregnant.' There's something very nurturing there, but I'm sure I have a glamorised view of pregnancy.

It hasn't seemed to have made any difference to David. Even when people ask him about it now, he says, 'Well, that's our birth story and it's the only story I know. It's just like my wife having a Caesarean rather than a vaginal delivery.' That's how important it is to us now. James's birth story is what it is—a light-hearted, warm, well thought-out, confident journey. And to us, it's a part of our history.

Postscript

Alison and David, who chose to use pseudonyms for this story, are still undecided about whether or not to try for another child using surrogacy. In 2002, Alison had her eggs frozen at an IVF clinic in Sydney in preparation, but they then changed their minds.

'The first time, it was like this driving passion to have a family,' says Alison, who lives with her family in inner-western Sydney. 'We would have sold the clothes off our backs. This time, we've got a family, we've got a house and it feels like there's a bit more to lose.'

While she says David would like more children, she is less willing to make the emotional and financial commitment. 'We had a bloody lucky run last time,' she says. 'I'd be in anguish. I'd be up in the middle of the night worrying about the fact we might not be able to feed James.'

Since James was born, the Australian government has introduced a law banning couples from taking frozen embryos out of the country, which would make having another child more difficult. Alison's sister has recently offered to be a surrogate for Alison, but for the moment she is keeping her eggs on ice. 'I've got everything I want,' she says. 'I'm healthy, I've got a job, and a happy family. What I'm not sure is that I want to roll the dice again.'

So much for a birth plan!

ZALI STEGGALL

It was 25 March 1998 and I'd just come back from the Nagano Winter Olympics, where I'd won bronze. I was sitting on the head table at a charity function in Sydney with all the older, important guests when I looked up towards another table and caught this guy's eye. *God, I'm never sitting on the right table with the nice-looking men,* I thought. *I'm always with the officials.* But not long after, the good-looking guy came over, introduced himself as David Cameron and sat down next to me.

I became absolutely flustered and had to ask for his name again. He was there as an Olympian too—he'd been to Atlanta in 1996—and said he was a rower. 'Do you paddle?' I asked. 'No, I row,' he said. He probably thought, *Oh, stupid blonde,* but we flirted through the night and I asked him to a do later in the week. It was actually the Manly mayor giving me the keys to Manly in front of 250 guests, and everyone who was remotely connected to me—family, friends, sponsors, school teachers—was there.

But the poor guy survived it all.

They say you subconsciously pick your mate as the person you'll make the best babies with and we were married a year and a half later when we were both 25.

I retired from skiing at the end of February 2002. I'd been competing internationally since I was 15, been to four Olympics, won the World Championships and although racing was still exciting, I was bored by all the in-between times. Dave and I wouldn't see each other for a couple of months at a time and I was travelling non-stop. I'd also always wanted to have one child before I was 30 or at least be on my way.

Initially, retirement was a pretty hard reality check. I'd had one job all my life and suddenly I had to start from scratch. I'd finished a BA in Communications and Media Studies from Griffith University while I was training and competing and I really wanted to see where that took me. But I found it frustrating. I was getting bits of TV work everywhere and while that probably would have been fine if I was 21 and willing to work at it, I was 28 and needed to have very set goals.

I was already starting to get restless after about six months of retirement and I'd always wanted to study law. The next term of the Legal Practitioners Admission Board course at Sydney University started in November, so I decided to enrol. And I figured, if I'm going to spend the next four years studying, I might as well get the babies out of the way. I also wanted to pack in as many things as I could to keep myself busy because I was missing skiing so much. So the pregnancy was very planned.

I'd been on the pill while competing—I couldn't exactly

afford accidents—and David and I went to Thredbo for a weekend and I'd forgotten to take them with me. We'd been talking about trying for kids, so I said, 'We might as well go off the pill and see how it goes.' We thought we would have heaps of time, but I conceived that first cycle. We were like 'Okay . . .!' but I wasn't really surprised. I trusted everything worked well with my body.

At six weeks I got my first sign of pregnancy—nausea. And unless I ate every three hours, even in the middle of the night, I'd feel sick and wake up cramped. But luckily that ended at eight weeks, just before I started uni.

I could only stomach savoury, salty, safe foods throughout the whole pregnancy. It was summer and I had this vision of eating heaps of fruit, vegetables and salads, but all I wanted to eat was pasta, Vegemite on toast and chips. I sometimes stopped at McDonald's on my way back from uni and thought, *What have I come to?*

So I spent my first summer in Australia in 13 years—I'd had 26 winters in a row—pregnant. And although it probably wasn't ideal being pregnant at the beach, it was quite good because January and February is the peak season on the world championship ski circuit. I'd constantly check the results on the Internet and my subconscious was obviously struggling because I kept having dreams about doing one more World Cup ski race. It was good to have the grounding fact that I was having a baby and I couldn't be selfish and just go back to sport very easily.

David and I took the hospital antenatal classes, I was doing Pilates and was also going to active birth classes held by Crows Nest physio JuJu Sundin, who was very much into the idea of empowerment in birth and doing everything you could before taking the drugs. Her philosophy was, 'Be physical, be active, and don't just lie around fighting the pain. Stomp, do whatever helps.'

I really didn't have set ideas about what I wanted the birth to be like nor was I really nervous. I tended to think I was fit, healthy, and had a reasonably good pain threshold. Women had been doing this for centuries and I was lucky to have so much help and technology on hand, but I thought I'd try and do it without drugs. I was also of the attitude that you couldn't control everything. You could only do the best you could in all circumstances and hope to rise to the challenge when it arrived.

Mum had my brother and me by Caesarean but I would have preferred a vaginal birth. Some people recover quickly from Caesareans but others don't. I knew they weren't always that straightforward and I also wanted to be up and around shortly after the birth. But I must admit, whenever anyone talked about episiotomies I'd think, *Oh God, I really wouldn't want that. I'd way prefer a Caesarean to that kind of stitching.*

I decided if I really did need drugs, then my game plan would be gas, pethidine and then epidural—only if really necessary. I definitely wasn't pro the epidural. I didn't like the idea of a needle in my spine and I was also really apprehensive about not feeling my body, as my physical presence had been such a big part of my life as an athlete.

All the books said I should write a birth plan, but when I asked my doctor about it a week before I was due he laughed. 'Just keep an open mind,' he said. 'You never know what's going to happen.'

Even though I had a pretty easy pregnancy, I was really sick of being pregnant towards the end. I had heartburn and I was huge. I was in maternity pants at 12 weeks—all my abs just let go. My target weight gain was 16 kilos and I held to it up until 38 weeks, but then the water retention started and I stopped counting. *Stuff this*, I thought. *I don't want to know any more.*

The baby was due on 23 May 2003, so I half-joked to my obstetrician, 'Right, book me in for an induction on the 24th.' But we waited.

I didn't have any major problems about being induced. I'm a practical person and didn't get hung up with the idea of 'I am woman and woman will control', or 'nature decides'. I'm against being told what the righteous way of doing things is and I certainly wasn't of the attitude that science and modern technology had to be kept out of it.

The baby was cooked by my due date and, according to my doctor, not undersized. He told me that the baby's head was engaged and my cervix was soft. There was also the health issue of the baby doing his first poo while still in the uterus if he was overdue. And admittedly, my new term at uni had started and my first assignment was due. I had actually hoped to go into labour the week before the due date so I could be back out before the term started.

I may have had selfish reasons for wanting to be induced, but I'm prepared to wear it. I'd always been in control of my life as an athlete and suddenly I wasn't and I just didn't want to wait any longer.

I went six days overdue and it was the longest week of my life. It was enough. But although I felt more than happy to be induced, I hesitated when my doctor told me that 80 per cent of induced women ended up with an epidural and a very high percentage of those ended as Caesareans. But we went ahead anyway.

So I went into hospital at Sydney's North Shore Private on the night of 28 May 2003. I'd had lots of Braxton Hicks contractions and was sure the prostaglandin gel, the first step of induction, would be enough for my body to do what it was meant to. But after the gel was put on my cervix that night nothing happened.

I probably got about five hours sleep and Dave came in at nine o'clock the next morning. They'd given me the gel again and I started to have really mild contractions but they were all over the place, so we started walking. And did we walk—we went up and down the hill in the hospital grounds, down to the carpark and back around the park. It must have been so obvious what we were trying to do—this big, waddling, pregnant woman walking all over the place.

By about 11.30 a.m. the contractions were becoming closer and more regular. I was finally in the early stages of labour and we were excited. 'Are you timing?' I asked Dave frantically as we stopped on the way back to the delivery suite.

At about one o'clock, the doctor checked my cervix and after discovering I'd started dilating, broke my waters. So there was no going back. We would have a baby by the end of the day.

I soon began having reasonable contractions on my own, which felt like severe period pain, mainly in my lower back. And my legs were becoming slightly cramped. I started walking around the room and bouncing up and down on the Swiss ball. The French Open was on TV and it was the perfect thing to watch because the point-scoring kept our attention while we counted down to the end of each contraction.

I had told Dave before I went into labour that he was going to be like my coach, pushing me along. But I think I turned into quite a demanding person. If he didn't start rubbing my back the second I told him to, I was like, 'Come on, what are you doing?'

But we were still joking with each other and things were going pretty well. I was being active. I had the ball. I was drinking my water. I had a bath, then a shower later and tried to relax. I was doing everything I'd been told to. And it was all helping.

At about three o'clock, the midwife came in to check my cervix again. 'You're about two centimetres,' she said. 'It hasn't really moved since we broke your waters.' I was devastated. I'd really expected things to have happened by then, and nothing had moved. Of course, if I hadn't been induced I would have still been at home at this stage and would probably only just have been thinking about coming into hospital. But you're on a quicker agenda once you're there. I understood that and was quite glad to get things moving along, too.

I was managing quite well, but because I was doing so many things to physically help bring on the labour and mentally cope with the pain, I soon became really, really tired. I was sitting on the Swiss ball and all of a sudden I thought, *Okay, sitting down feels really good*. I just didn't have the desire to stomp around any more. And that's probably where JuJu would have said that I really needed to get moving.

I wanted the midwife to check my cervix again, but she was reluctant to. She was putting it off because she knew she wasn't going to have good news. But I was insistent. At five o'clock she checked and I was only three centimetres dilated, seven centimetres from my target. 'You're kidding, aren't you?' I said, completely discouraged. Nobody had told me just how disheartening that could be.

The midwife told me they were going to have to give me the oxytocin drip to get the contractions going. I didn't really want it, but it was obvious by then I didn't have a choice. I asked them to set up the gas because I knew the drip was going to be hard work. I also figured I would be in control of the gas and could take small amounts of it when I needed.

As soon as they put the drip in, I felt the oxytocin working. 'Here we go,' I said, and all of a sudden everything kicked into second gear—the contractions were coming harder and faster—and I was finding it a lot harder to cope.

I had the needle in my arm and I could still have done the jumping around, but I didn't. I'd sat on that ball for too long and my legs had stiffened and become really sore and cramped. I was okay mentally but physically I was resisting the contractions instead of working with them. There was no way I could move around to get those endorphins flowing. I was just too tired to do it any more.

The midwives quickly upped the dose and by around seven o'clock, they'd cranked the drip level right up and I started to feel nauseous from the gas. And it didn't take long before I switched on to what that meant—if the gas made me sick, then I'd have to stop taking it, which meant all of a sudden I'd have no painkiller when the next contraction hit.

'Right, I need something else here,' I said. 'What's my next option? Where's the pethidine?' By then I had a different midwife and she told me I couldn't have pethidine. I'm not sure why but all I heard was, 'No pethidine.'

A friend had told me that after a certain time the hospital's anaesthetist would go on night duty, which meant it would take longer to get hold of one. And it was getting late. So I thought if I was going to end up needing an epidural, and realistically I probably would, then I might as well do it now rather than wait two hours.

'How long would it take to get someone for the epidural?' I asked between contractions. 'We can have someone up in five minutes,' the midwife said.

I decided to see how far along I was, so they got me up on the bed and I was four centimetres dilated. Unbelievable. I thought at that rate it was going to take hours, and I asked them to send up the anaesthetist right away.

Just as I was asking for the epidural, I vomited. And while I was being sick over the bed without the gas, I got hit by a contraction. And then my body went into one big cramp—it was as if every muscle had gone into overdrive all at once. Forget the 'relaxing to go along with the experience'. I felt like I couldn't do anything. I couldn't even move my legs.

Everything seemed to have avalanched within minutes—we were quite in control and then all of a sudden it all took over. I could see Dave starting to look worried and I squeezed his hand, looked into his eyes and cried, 'Where is the epidural?'

The anaesthetist arrived really quickly—the hospital was great—but because I'd been so sure I wasn't going to need an epidural I hadn't filled out any forms. So there the doctor was, saying, 'You understand there's a chance of one in 10 000 you might have mild paralysis and blah blah blah.' And there I was with vomit down my face saying, 'Just do it. I don't care.'

People are often scared about the epidural needle hurting. I didn't feel a thing. One second I was cramped and in agony and the next I had this warm flow over my body. No kidding, it was bliss. And then everything went calm. The storm was over and I finally relaxed. I was so comfortable that mentally I could handle anything. I could actually think again because my mind wasn't busy coping with the next contraction.

I had another examination and amazingly, I had dilated to nine plus centimetres. The minute they gave me that epidural, my muscles relaxed and bang, they stopped fighting the contractions.

I was now feeling pretty good. 'I'm nine plus,' I said. 'I'm calm, I've got the epidural. We can move on.' But my midwife thought differently, as the baby's heart rate had gone right up while I was vomiting. 'No dear, you don't understand,' she said. 'Your baby is distressed when the oxytocin is on, so we've turned it off and you don't have enough contractions. We've called your doctor and we're prepping you for a Caesarean.'

I couldn't believe it. It felt like the last straw. I'd already had all the drugs I had hoped to avoid, been through a fair share of labour and for some reason, right then, I really didn't want to have a Caesarean. And it wasn't because of a feeling that I'd failed, or that to be a true woman I had to experience a natural birth. I was just peeved I hadn't quite managed to get through the whole thing the way I thought I would.

And then my doctor arrived, as cool as a cucumber. 'I see it's all been happening here,' he said with a laugh. By that stage I was still having mild contractions, but the baby's head had come back up. I told him I still really wanted a vaginal delivery. He said he'd prepare me for a Caesarean, take me down to the operating theatre and if the baby's head became engaged by the time we were there, we could give it a go. 'It's your choice,' he said.

It took about half an hour to get me ready and they wheeled me down to the operating theatre. 'This is the biggest dose of drugs I've had in my life,' I joked with the anaesthetist, who had just topped up the epidural for the Caesarean. 'I've had no injuries in 23 years of skiing, so I'm just having all the drugs today.'

Dave, who was now getting used to the idea of a Caesarean, went in to get ready for theatre while I lay in there. And then, at the last minute, after everyone had gowned up, my doctor said, 'The head's engaged. You've still got contractions, we can give it a go.' I said, 'Right,' and they rushed out to get Dave.

So there I was, in an operating theatre with my feet up in elastic-band stirrups. And I had the full crowd—a paediatrician, my doctor, his assistant, the anaesthetist, another assistant and a couple of nurses plus Dave. I actually was kind of regretting I was totally lucid. So much for a birthing plan and any hope of keeping some decorum.

At first, my doctor tried the suction cap. I couldn't feel much so somebody felt my tummy to tell me when the next contraction was and told me when to push. I actually had to visualise pushing, but it was helping.

My baby was halfway down the birth canal, but the cap wasn't working. So my doctor said he was going to use forceps, or what Dave called later the 'massive salad servers', which meant I had to have an episiotomy. But it didn't really bother me one way or the other by then. I was busy focusing on pushing and trying to do the best I could for all that I was in control of.

And then at 9.05 p.m. they pulled my baby out, quickly showed him to me and whisked him away. I don't think he was breathing at the time but in a few seconds there was crying. Everything kicked into gear and they told me he was a boy. They wrapped him up, brought him back to me and we rubbed noses, an Eskimo kiss, and they took him away again. And then my doctor stitched me back up. I didn't care. It wasn't the end of the world. I was just happy that my baby was fine and I was fine.

The epidural level was still quite high and as I was talking to the nurse, my cheeks began to feel numb and tingly. And that's not supposed to happen. So suddenly the concern shifted to me. I could stop breathing if the epidural went too high.

They quickly gave me some adrenalin to lower the levels and everything went a bit blurry. I think the drama of the last hour suddenly hit me and I went into shock. They kept me in observation and my doctor told Dave it was probably best he went with the baby, who we'd named Rex, rather than with me as I was going to be in ga-ga land for a while. He didn't want to leave but told me later that he figured if I was in a bad way I was in the right place, so he went with Rex.

They told me that the comedown from the epidural would be a bit nasty and they were right. It really was one of the weirdest experiences. I was lying in observation with all these people coming out of operations and I had absolutely no feeling in any part of my body. I was numb from the neck down. It was surreal. I was lying there surprised that I'd had a boy because I really thought I was having a girl, and at the same time I had uncontrollable trembling.

The nurses were putting ice cubes on my skin to check where I had feeling and I knew they would be satisfied once I could feel below my ribs. I could sense the feeling coming back after an hour or so and I really wanted to get back to see Rex, so I might have exaggerated a little bit. But they were on to me. 'Now this is important,' the nurse said. 'You just can't say, "Yes, I can feel that."'

I really wanted to know Rex was okay, so they eventually took me back upstairs to the delivery ward. I was on oxygen and I think my poor parents got a shock. They gave Rex to me and by the time he had finished his first breastfeed my toes were tingling. I felt fine but very tired and Dave left at about one o'clock in the morning.

I was on oxygen that night as a precaution and they brought Rex in at about seven o'clock in the morning. My doctor had wisely advised me to get up and have a shower, get dressed and do all the normal things, as I wasn't sick. So I had a shower, which felt so good, and right then I was glad I hadn't had a Caesarean. For all the other stitches, I was happy I could be up and about and was not immobilised.

I spent that first day just staring at Rex. I was entranced. I'd only just met this person and his features were completely new to me, yet he looked so familiar. It was as if I'd always known him. 'It was you hiding in there,' I kept saying.

But he really looked like he'd struggled his way through birth. He looked like a boxer. His right eye was all swollen, his head was red from the cap and he had a little scratch above his eye from the forceps because his head was crooked coming down the birth canal. All I could say was, 'You poor little fella.' But from day one he was fine and today he's a very contented little boy. His birth may have been traumatic, but everything since has all been very calm. He has been a great eater and sleeper the whole way through.

I was so glad I had the doctor I had. I don't think many doctors like using forceps and a lot would have gone straight to a Caesarean. And if I'd had the Caesarean, I would probably have had to have one for my second baby. In the end it was all good. Rex came out happy and healthy and I still had the option for number two. My only regret is that I wish someone had told me sooner about those blow-up rings you can sit on while learning to breastfeed—sitting on those episiotomy stitches for long periods was agony. But a swim a few weeks later down at Manly on a cool, crisp day did the world of good.

A lot of people would be disappointed with the birth experience I had and I think people thought I was going to be negative. But I didn't expect birth to be straightforward and it honestly went the way I expected. And having quite an intervened birth doesn't make it less mine or less empowering. It was definitely a success to me.

If I went back I'd probably do a few things differently—I'd take the pethidine and not the gas to avoid the nausea, or possibly go for the epidural from the beginning. But I would still have been induced. I mean he had a 38 centimetre head circumference and was nine pounds.

I don't really think much about the birth today. The whole thing was just a part of the process for Dave and me. It was only the beginning. It was an amazing experience, but Rex is the truly amazing thing. And unlike sporting successes where the high is over so quickly, he keeps on being more amazing every day.

Postscript

Four days after coming home from hospital with Rex Steggall Cameron, Zali returned to uni and managed to get her assignment in on time. 'It was the best thing for me mentally,' she says. 'Life still goes on and I was quite happy to have those couple of hours away. And both Dave and Rex love their boys' nights.'

Zali is certain that Rex, who she says is 'chubby, but has really wide shoulders', will take after his parents and 'be quite a good athlete'. At just nine weeks old, he was given his first taste of his mother's preferred sport when Zali popped him in a pouch and took him for a run at the Thredbo ski fields. 'Everyone was horrified,' she recalls with a laugh. 'But I was very careful.'

Zali continues to work part time at her father's law

practice, is still studying law and plans to be pregnant with the couple's second child in early 2005. She hopes he or she will arrive in late September, as exams start earlier that month. But whenever the baby is born, he or she will have a busy time ahead. 'Sport's great for keeping kids focused and busy,' she says. 'You get 'em tired, so there's no way they've got the energy for trouble. I think that is going to be my motto.'

'The greatest high I had ever experienced'

LIZ SCOTT

I grew up in Melbourne and Adelaide, spent most of my twenties in Adelaide and Sydney and moved to Alice Springs when I was 28. I had a long-term relationship with someone in the Northern Territory and then Sydney, but he didn't want children as he'd already had three when he was younger.

I always knew I wanted children. I felt it was part of my life's script, and started feeling resentful towards him. Friends kept saying, 'Just get pregnant,' but I was really in love and knew how he felt. That seemed out of the question and I decided to leave him. Everyone said, 'You can't leave. You're in love. Work it out.' But I knew having children was a very important part of who I was.

me inheritance left from my mother, who had
rlier, so I decided to see the world while
out. I started in Russia—possibly so I
him—and then went to England and

I came back to Australia two years later, in March 1994, and tried settling in Adelaide, but couldn't. I returned to Alice, quite unsure of what I was doing with my life. But when the plane touched down on the tarmac, I thought, *I'm home*, and burst into tears.

I went to a party that first weekend back in town and met Michael. We started a light, enjoyable relationship with me feeling good, as he was the first lover I'd had where my ex didn't come between us on the pillow.

It was a fairly casual thing for the first six months, but people were telling me 'Don't go near him. Use contraception. He's a walking sperm bank.' He'd already had three children to three different mothers. Did I listen? No.

I'd had an extremely regular menstrual cycle since I was ten and was very conscientious about contraception. But one night after we had an intense love-making session, Michael went to sleep and I started having very weird feelings in my pelvis. It was six days before I was due to ovulate—I had never used contraception at that stage in my cycle before because it had always been safe—and my pelvis and abdomen became really hot. I started having very strange thoughts and visions. It was as if I was either very stoned or in a deep meditation.

I kept seeing an image of a pink and yellow lotus flower unfolding with layers and more layers of petals opening up. I had these esoteric thoughts floating through me and all the while my pelvis was getting hotter and hotter and hotter. *I've just conceived a bloody baby*, I thought.

I woke Michael up after a couple of hours and asked him to feel my belly. 'Oh fuck,' he said. 'It's burning hot.'

I knew I was pregnant. And the next morning, the smell of coffee made me throw up and I stopped smoking cigarettes immediately.

Then it went from unplanned pregnancy to unplanned situation.

I'd always had this fantasy, like most people I suppose, of having kids when I was in a fairly loving and committed relationship and I didn't necessarily know if I wanted to commit to Michael, or he to me. I thought it would also be unfair on the child if the relationship was dictated by the pregnancy.

Initially, I refused to move in with him and spent the first three months going, 'Oh dear, oh dear.' But there was never a thought of a termination and Michael and I soon began living together.

I was going to be 37 when I had the baby, so I was old, overweight and unfit. I had many of the problematic ticks but I had a fantastic GP. He knew I had a good relationship with my body and was into alternative health and asked me if I had considered a home birth.

I was very drawn to the idea, but Michael was reluctant. He was mainly against it because it cost money—$1200— and it meant taking a very different responsibility towards the baby and the birth and I guess a different level of commitment to the pregnancy.

My GP said that as far as he was concerned I was medically very healthy, and being older just meant I was going to get tired. He also said I had to be careful as overweight women often ballooned during pregnancy. But I was vomiting 24 hours a day for the first three months—whoever labelled it morning sickness had a sense of humour and must have been a man—and with care I actually lost weight during the pregnancy.

My doctor did ask me about the birthing history in my family and I lied. It's absolutely shocking. My mother was in labour for four days with one baby and two for another, and my sister was in labour for three days and had a very interventionist and traumatic birth with her son.

I could be wrong, but I think much of that had to do with fear. My family culture was very fear-oriented. There were a lot of absent emotions, a lot of abuse. So knowing that the medical model was based on the fear of what could go wrong, I decided early on that if no one knew they needed to be fearful then they wouldn't be. So I didn't tell anyone, including Michael.

I saw my GP regularly because he was my ideal birthing practitioner and every now and then he'd say, 'Have you thought any more about the home birth?' He was still really encouraging. But as Michael was so resistant to the idea, I reluctantly agreed to go to the midwives' clinic that was attached to the local hospital. I left it as late as possible, when I was 20 weeks.

I soon discovered that there was a real difference between the attitudes of the midwives and my GP, and I started to get a little concerned. The baby was really quite large, and when I went to the clinic and they found out I'd actually lost weight, they started getting worried. My GP had warned me that the hospital really hit the panic button when a woman births for the first time at 37, and when the midwives said they were going to keep a close watch on me I was like, 'There's no need. It's all fine.'

I loved being pregnant. I glowed, looked fabulous and

felt fabulous and I was much more relaxed than the midwives were.

A lot of people were also saying, 'You're 37, you'd better have an amniocentesis.' But after discussing it with my GP, Michael and I decided against doing the test. Our decision was based on whether or not I would have a termination on finding something out, and I really thought I wouldn't. I also thought, *Why on earth would you do something that risks the baby's life*? And there was a risk. Perhaps if there was no risk to the baby, it might have been a different choice.

I really hated going to see the midwives unless I got a couple of the ones I liked, and I also hated going to the hospital. My stress levels would go up and I could feel fear coming in. Maybe it was a fear of losing control of my pregnancy, but I also hated the stories I kept hearing about people giving birth in the hospital with lots of intervention.

And I didn't like the hospital's guidelines that restricted what type of birth I could have. I had a real sense I might want a water-birth, as water really pacifies me and there were other benefits such as pain relief and stretchability. It wasn't a desperate desire that my baby should 'move from internal fluid to external fluid' to make its entry into the world gentler. It was more about me and my needs. And it made sense.

So then it became an issue. 'What if I want a water-birth?' 'Well, you're not allowed a water-birth.' 'Why not?' 'Oh, don't be bloody difficult, you're not allowed it.' 'Why not?'

As I got further into my pregnancy, the baby got bigger and bigger, and at about 30 weeks the midwives said they needed me to have fortnightly ultrasounds. But as far as I was concerned, the previous ultrasound had shown everything was fine and we didn't need any more.

So then I had to sign a refusal of medical treatment form. And they made me sign a new one every two weeks when I went there. I was giving them the shits.

At my 36-week appointment, I picked up my case notes when the midwife left the room—I used to be a nurse—and there, written in big red writing, was 'Likely Caesarean'. I was outraged. I went home and immediately started talking home birth again. Michael still had real concerns, so everything was up in the air.

I was in despair. I really needed Michael's support. I also wanted everything to be clear and clean between us before the birth, wherever it was. I had a feeling that during my labour I would go very inward and not communicate with anybody, so he was to be my buffer against the outside world. I needed to be able to look into his eyes and feel complete clarity and trust. I also had a strong belief that the more shit I sorted out before the birth, the better labour I would have.

I said to him one night that I thought there were some untruths between us, and of course, out came a story about an affair—prior to our time together, but which had big implications for me in this small town.

It sent me into a spiral. I became a complete screaming emotional mess, and drove across town to a friend's house. I basically went stark raving mad and became really concerned for the baby. I couldn't think of who to ring, so I rang the town's independent midwife, who I knew socially. She came over, sat with me for six hours and encouraged me to deal with all my emotional stuff. At the end of that I thought, *Well, that's it. There is no longer a safe choice. I have to have a home birth with her.*

She had a really good relationship with my GP and after speaking with him and understanding that I wanted the option of a water-birth, she agreed to do it. I was 38 weeks pregnant.

But there were all sorts of issues. She hadn't followed me through the pregnancy and she also had three other women due in the same week, including her usual home birth assistant. So I was her last priority.

I stayed away from Michael for four days, processing my stuff and being nurtured by friends. I soon felt that I was in charge of this birth and he had lost some of his rights. I told him what I'd decided and that I had agreed with the midwife that if she wasn't happy with what was happening at home, I was prepared to go to hospital to deliver. But I knew I wasn't going to. I'd never been so clear about anything before in my life.

It was early January 1996, and we were in a heat wave. I had this really strong sense I was going to go into labour the next day, which was the day before my due date. So the first thing I had to do was set up the home birth labour pool—a round, old-fashioned Clark's style rubber one about two feet deep and six feet in diameter. We rang the woman who was the first cab due off the home birth rank to see how she was going and fortunately she didn't think she was anywhere near labour. The pool was still boxed, so we went and collected it from her on the proviso that if she or either of the other women went into labour and wanted it, it had to be emptied and sent over immediately, no matter what my situation was.

Michael and my stepson set the pool up on the back verandah. We had a great backyard beyond the pergola, which housed a lovely garden edged by a beautiful pond filled with lotus lilies, just like the ones I saw the night the baby was conceived. There was also a rockery waterfall where the recycled pond water flowed down back into the pond. I had a very romantic vision of me birthing in the pool by the pond in the middle of the night, with candles everywhere and the water going.

I spent the next day very relaxed, setting up candles through the verandah garden and pottering around. As a gesture of love, Michael killed one of our chooks and cooked up a soup for me, for after the birth. But the very smell of it cooking brought back the fabulous old morning sickness.

At about eight o'clock that night, I started feeling peculiar. Really odd. Michael kept asking if I was having Braxton Hicks contractions or if I was in labour. 'How on earth do I know?' I said. 'I haven't done this before.' But I knew it was the real thing, based on nothing but intuition. And then the pains got more and more serious.

I had always considered myself to have a fairly high pain threshold but this was shocking, so I told Michael to ring the midwife. She arrived, took one look at me and said, 'Oh for God's sake, don't ring me again for period pain.' 'Fucking period pain,' I said. 'Let me assure you, this is not period pain.' Her reply? 'Just go to bed and get some sleep.'

Get some sleep? I couldn't even lie down. I couldn't do anything but crawl around on all fours. Eventually she came back, but was still unconvinced. 'This is what I would classify as early contractions,' she said. I was on the floor, leaning against the coffee table, telling her she needed to take me seriously. She didn't, and went home again. But before she left she asked if we had let the neighbours know about the birth, so Michael went and told them that if they heard any noises, not to ring the cops. I was just having a baby.

By around 11 p.m. my contractions were five minutes apart, I was in severe pain, crawling on my hands and knees down the hallway through vomit and totally wanting to push. And I thought I was going to start shitting—my biggest paranoia about giving birth—or prolapsing my entire innards.

When the midwife left, I got Michael to call our support person, Louise, and even though I was told not to, I just went and got in that pool. I didn't give a rat about anybody else. I had the candles lit everywhere and I stayed in that pool the whole time and it was fantastic.

The contractions were unbelievable but the pool gave me great relief. I was buoyant and my whole body weight was supported. I couldn't squat for ten minutes on dry land. In the pool, I squatted for hours. Occasionally I would lean over this beanbag type pool toy, but most of the time I just squatted. And by about two o'clock in the morning the midwife returned and saw that it was a bit serious.

I really felt like I was managing the pain despite it being so intense. I went very inward, as I suspected I would, into a very deep meditation. I was facing the waterfall and the pond throughout the entire labour, and once I was there I was very conscious of the water cycle, going from the pond, up through the waterfall, down into the pond and up again. I went into this mantra for about ten hours of 'Let good, let go' or 'Let God, let go'—and I'm not a religious person.

When it really started to hurt and I felt scared, I'd make myself find something to love, and at times that was a real struggle. Sometimes it was the goldfish, other times it was the baby.

I was loud. I was like a bear growling, a tiger roaring, and the sound came from a very deep place. And I didn't want to talk to anyone. It was as though there was this veil between me and the world and I wanted to stay in that place. The midwife asked me something at one stage and it just irritated me. I didn't want to talk, so I didn't. 'She's losing it. She's not responding, we'll have to take her to the hospital,' she said to Michael after a while. And I just went, 'Would you fuck off and leave me be? I'm fine.'

I didn't get a kick out of the pain, but I loved climbing above it. Not being a sporty person, I'd never experienced that endorphin rush people talk about.

And at some point during the night, after hours and hours of pain, I got this incredibly stoned feeling. It was as if someone was injecting me with a drug, or I was getting a pump of pain relief, every third contraction. It was amazing and I really got a buzz out of it. I knew that all I had to do was get through three contractions and it would kick in again. It was like pain control and I was so excited that I was doing this. I was using my will and inner strength to rise above the pain and not handing my power over to anyone or anything else. It was the greatest high I had ever experienced.

I could feel my whole body opening up. And I could

see it all happening, even though I was often doubled over during contractions. I'd watch them and loved seeing my body rippling down in a very snake-esque way.

Daylight came, and every now and then the midwife said I was too relaxed and it was slowing down the labour, so they'd put a sarong around me and make me walk around the yard. At one stage, I looked up and saw someone looking over from a balcony at the motel which backed on to our yard. *Who gives a rat*, I thought.

But being out of the pool was sheer hell and I'd always take the shortest way back. All I wanted to do was be in that pool.

The pain was extraordinary, and around this time I heard the midwife whisper to Michael, 'I think the baby's posterior.' And I came out of my little veil and said, 'So does that mean I'm not a wimp after all?' The baby was completely locked in my spine and that's why I had been pushing all the time and that's why it had been so painful. *Oh God*, I thought, *how much longer can I keep this up?*

It was nine o'clock and the beginnings of a new day of heat wave. All the candles had melted away and Michael had to put blankets over the shadecloth above the verandah and hose it down to try and keep it cool.

About an hour later, the baby finally started to enter the birth canal, but I couldn't get it out. And of course, I pooed. It was my one great fear, and there was my poor birth assistant catching the poo with our vegetable strainer. And I laughed.

After two hours of pushing I told the midwife, 'It's like something's stuck over the baby's head and it won't come out.' So she gently put her hand inside—I can still feel the sensation—and my cervix had capped over the baby's head and caught on its nose. She peeled it back off its head, which made it a lot easier. I am sure the baby would have been dragged out with forceps if we were in the hospital.

But it was still a really hard time. I had been pushing for 13 hours, it was now 47 degrees and I was physically exhausted. My whole body hurt.

And then finally, as I leant over the side of the pool, my baby popped out. My waters hadn't broken, so he came out in his vortex bag and as I leant back, I could see his face through the bag and pool water, which they'd been sterilising with salt. His little head burst through the bag and I let him cruise around the pool because I didn't want to know the sex straight away—I just wanted a moment with this baby without any expectation or identity. I felt completely elated and so powerful and able.

As with all water-births, there was quite a lot of blood in the pool. I pulled my new baby up and out of the water to cuddle and have a look at him, and straight away realised his umbilical cord had snapped. There were no instruments nearby, as I hadn't wanted the cord to be cut until it had stopped pulsating, which would have normally taken about an hour.

Suddenly there was panic. They couldn't tell how much of the blood in the pool was his or mine, but I was pretty laid back and telling everyone to calm down. I was just so thrilled with myself, the baby and the universe. I thought I could conquer the world.

Michael pinched the cord with his fingers while the midwife and Louise frantically tried to find the clamp. Someone soon found it and the midwife talked me into letting her take a bit of blood from the baby to do an emergency haemoglobin check at the hospital, and he was fine. Later, we worked out I must have had a short umbilical cord and probably lifted him a bit too high from the water. A similar thing happened with my second baby, but that time we were prepared.

They asked me to get out of the pool and I got onto our bed to deliver the placenta. No one had told me how painful delivering the placenta would be. It wasn't coming out so my midwife, who was keen to check it because of the cord, tugged on it. It seriously hurt and contractions started again. *You've got to be kidding*, I thought. *I've just done 13 hours of hard labour*. But it eventually came out.

Our baby was very, very alert. He was 4.1 kilos with a really cone-shaped head. He looked like something out of *The Coneheads* because he had been in the birth canal for so long. And although he was very big, I didn't tear at all due to being in the water for so long. The skin just stretched.

After the placenta was delivered, I had a shower and came back into our bedroom to find Michael and our new baby son sitting up watching the cricket on television. Michael said he wanted a name that could lead the Australian XI onto Lords. And what does Harry want to be? The captain of the Australian cricket team.

Postscript

Liz gave birth to her second son, Zac, in the home birth pool in hospital on 1 November 1997. 'I had a Clayton's— the home birth you have when you're not having a home birth,' she says. 'Harry was only 21 months old and I felt I would be looking after two babies, Harry and the unborn one, if I was at home.'

She says her second non-posterior birth was 'easy-schmeemy' compared with the first. 'When I had my first contraction with Zac, I thought "Oh, this is what a normal contraction's like",' she recalls. 'Now I know why they told me to have a lie down.'

Liz and Michael married in 1997 and separated in 2001 and Liz remains a full-time mum. 'I adore the boys,' she says. 'We just sit and laugh. They're a different species.'

Since having the boys, Liz has become a health consumer advocate and sits on various medical boards. She says she is keen to steer the medical profession away from the view that birth is a medical problem that needs fixing and requires 'crisis intervention' and to work towards a system which gives women more control and continuity of care. 'I wish all women felt confident and empowered in giving birth,' she says. 'Then, if they did end up having intervention of one sort or another, they would probably not have as much grief around them.'

For Liz, her biggest grief is that she will not give birth again. 'I wish I had started earlier,' she says. 'I feel an incredible sense of self-knowing and self-assurance when I give birth. I just wish I could harness that more in my everyday life. It is such a good anchor.'

'I thought I was risking my baby's life'

KATRINA O'BRIEN

It wasn't long after I gave up breastfeeding Joe that I found I was pregnant again. It must have been really early on, as the blue lines on the pregnancy test were incredibly faint. Of course, I made Fabio go out and buy a couple more tests to check, and got the same result before deciding to go to the doctor. When I got there I did another wee test which came back negative. I had a blood test anyway, and indeed I was.

Fabio and I were thrilled but it seemed to happen really quickly. It took us a while with Joe. I'd been off the pill for about a year all up, although it was probably only seven months of serious trying. This time it was two periods and we were there.

The strange thing was I didn't feel pregnant at all. I felt really well. I was incredibly sick for about half the pregnancy with Joe. I used to have a going-home-from-work vomit in the car at around Edgecliff station every night, and back then I'd made Fabio get rid of all these placemats we'd bought from a recent trip to Bali. Seeing them reminded me of the spicy food we'd eaten there, and even the thought made me want to throw up. I certainly knew I was pregnant a couple of weeks later though, when the all-day nausea returned.

I talked a little bit about what I wanted to do for the birth this time on my first visit with my obstetrician. He looked at the card from my previous pregnancy and birth and said it was probably likely I'd have to have another Caesarean. There was always a risk the scar might burst if a woman has a vaginal delivery second time around, he told me.

He was reading my old records and saying how my cervix hadn't dilated after ten hours of labour. It was quite wrong—I'd probably only had about five hours all up—and funnily enough I had to remind him that he wasn't actually there for Joe's birth. He was away on holiday and his stand-in did the deed. He said he'd check his notes, but he was very good and after I told him I had an inkling I wanted to try for a vaginal delivery, he didn't rule it out.

Joe had been born on 7 December 1999 by emergency Caesarean. He was a week overdue and after being induced the night before—a procedure I didn't want but was encouraged to have—his heartbeat dropped dramatically. By the time it was decided he needed to be born quickly, I was lying on my side to make sure his heart kept beating.

It was all terribly scary. I was swamped by a mass of medical staff who put in tubes, needles and a catheter and it felt as though my body had become a birthing vessel and I was an extra on a hospital soapie. I was wheeled down to theatre, stunned and tired and more than a little concerned. 'I can still feel my legs,' I kept saying to anyone who'd listen. The anaesthetist reassured me all would be fine and numb—it was—and Fabio was just as bewildered. I later discovered he was found wandering around the theatre without a mask on.

Having a Caesarean for Joe was not totally unexpected. It was discovered on my second ultrasound that my placenta was right over my cervix—not the most convenient spot—which meant it was unlikely I'd deliver vaginally. I used to sit in those prenatal classes with Fabio feeling slightly sad but resigned to the fact that I was going to have a Caesar. Hell, I probably wouldn't have survived childbirth if it was 100 years ago, so I was pretty okay with the option.

Then, at 36 weeks, I had another ultrasound and my placenta had moved to where it was supposed to be. So suddenly I was all clear for a natural birth and that's when I started taking those birth books a little more seriously.

I didn't love having a Caesarean, but I didn't mind either. I was just so ecstatic when I saw my chubby, 3.8 kilo baby boy, screaming with the most gorgeously huge mouth over that flimsy green curtain. It could have been the pethidine—some people hate the sensation of it running through their veins, I thought it was quite pleasant—but I was blissed out for days afterwards. For all my angst before I was induced, I really couldn't have cared less how he was born as long as he was okay.

The second time around was different. As the pregnancy progressed, it was becoming more and more likely I'd have to have a Caesarean. The baby was not engaged, my cervix was far from ripe and I was approaching my due date, which bizarrely was Joe's second birthday. And once you have had a C-section, my doctor told me that being induced was out of the question, as there was just too much risk. I could sense he was thinking Caesar and I found myself getting quite strung out.

The decision to have a Caesarean for Joe's birth had been out of my control: I did it because I had to. With an elective one, even though my doctor was telling me it was the only choice, I felt like it was going to be more like an operation than a birth. I also started to feel terribly uneasy about the idea of someone cutting through my uterus again. And although I recovered well after the birth last time, I wasn't looking forward to not being able to run around after Joe for a while. I also had some kind of earth-mother desire to purge my baby out the way it was meant to.

But there was an upside to having a Caesarean. Some women absolutely hate staying in hospital. I love it. I love being in my own room with my newborn, having my own phone line and TV and especially having meals and morning and afternoon tea delivered to my door. To me it was like a little holiday, a break from reality, and the good thing about a Caesar was that you got to stay in hospital for a week rather than just four days.

As my due day passed—no surprises there—I went to my last regular appointment with my obstetrician. He gave me an internal. 'Your cervix is still hard,' he said, 'and the baby's not engaged.'

We still hadn't really talked in detail about what we were going to do for the birth. I was somehow still hopeful for a vaginal delivery and really wanted to give my body more time. My doctor was very patient and agreed that if I went into spontaneous labour over the next few days, I could give it a go. If I didn't, then the Caesar was booked for Wednesday, 12 December 2001.

I also asked for one last appointment on the day before the Caesarean—my sister had told me those internals could sometimes get things moving—and he agreed. But it was looking highly unlikely that I was ever going to give birth naturally, and I sobbed uncontrollably under the shower when I got home.

I had been having a bit of vaginal discharge, but really thought nothing of it. Then, over that weekend, I felt this great big *gloop*, and when I went to the bathroom it looked like a small jellyfish had escaped. I became a bit excited but all the birthing books said labour could still be a week away, if this was indeed that mysterious thing called a show.

The three of us had a lovely weekend and when the day before C-day arrived Joe, Fabio and I went to the beach for a walk. I stood there and looked down at my boys playing on the sand and thought how strange it was that we could be this amazingly tight threesome one day and then the next we would be four. I went for a brisk walk along the promenade, barefoot and huge in a sarong and T-shirt, and did as many yoga poses as I could in public. I felt good and was really willing my body to do something.

I couldn't wait to tell my obstetrician about the plug at my 10.30 a.m. appointment, but after he checked my cervix again he found it to be still rock hard. Depressing. 'So some women just don't go into labour?' I asked him as graciously as possible. 'Yes,' he replied, and gave me an operation consent form to fill out and told me the anaesthetist would give me a call later that afternoon.

And so it wasn't to be. Fabio went to work and I went home with Joe, resigned to the fact that the next day I would be having the Caesarean, yet excited that I would soon see my baby. But I was really quite unprepared: I hadn't packed a thing, had washing on the line and was expecting a Coles Online grocery delivery between 4 and 6 p.m.

After putting Joe to bed for his afternoon nap, I stuffed myself with a felafel roll and chips and decided to have a little lie down. And then I suddenly felt it—something like a sharp constipation cramp. Even though I'd been in labour before, it had been induced. That was hard, fast and like having your body dragged behind a truck, so I really didn't know what to expect now.

I got up to take the clothes off the line—I'd read somewhere that if you walked around and the pangs went away, then you weren't in labour, or was it the other way around? I tried both ways and they still kept coming.

At 1.46 p.m, I started timing the cramps on Joe's Thomas the Tank Engine watch. I called my sister and a friend to get their opinion on whether or not I was in labour—they reckoned I was and were more excited than I was—and then called Fabio, who didn't believe me. 'But you're booked in for a Caesarean tomorrow,' he kept saying. 'You can't be.'

Even though he understood my absolute desire was to have a vaginal delivery, I knew Fabio was secretly relieved I was to have a Caesar. We'd done that one before and he doesn't like surprises. I hung up the phone but the pains didn't go away and after timing them—they were about five minutes apart—I called him back and told him to come home.

I was so excited but I was getting a bit flustered between contractions, thinking about poor little Joe, what to pack—CDs? Lollies? Sparkly pink thongs?—getting the clothes off the line, and the Coles delivery.

As I danced around the apartment thinking I was superwoman, the anaesthetist called. 'I think I'm in the early stages of labour,' I told him. He didn't sound as thrilled as I was and continued to say things like, 'Well, you can really only have a glass of juice or a cup of tea before coming into the hospital in the morning.' It was the oddest conversation—it was as if he was ignoring everything I said.

I didn't know whether to stay home or go to the hospital, so I rang the delivery suite. 'I'm booked in for a Caesarean tomorrow morning,' I told the midwife, trying to contain my excitement. 'But I'm in labour and the contractions are about five minutes apart.' She thought it best to come in.

Mum soon arrived—it's a very strange thing to have contractions in front of your mother—and then the non-believing husband turned up in a slight tizz. I had a shower and little Joe woke up.

There's a photo of the three of us crouched down on our front steps, taken moments before I left for hospital. My hair's shower-damp and I'm beaming down at the camera with Joe smiling beside my bump. The pains were getting longer and stronger, but I was just so happy that my body had decided to go into labour by itself.

After the 10-minute seatbelt-grasping drive to the hospital, I was led to the labour ward. The midwife who I'd spoken to on the phone told us to get comfortable. 'Your doctor knows you're here and the anaesthetist is on his way to have a chat,' she said. I thought that was quite strange—I'd heard private hospitals were renowned for high epidural rates, but had no idea drugs would arrive without even asking for them. I was also feeling like I didn't really need them—yet.

I was doing my best to breathe and sway through the contractions and not long after, the anaesthetist made his entrance. After introducing himself and asking me to sit down as if I was in his office rather than him in my labour room—I stood—he started talking about squeezing us in for a Caesarean that night as if we were some big inconvenience. And I suddenly realised he wasn't there to offer pain relief.

I started to panic. Didn't he know going into spontaneous labour was the best thing that could have happened? Wasn't everything going to run smoothly now—no operation, no cuts and catheters, no pubic-hair shaves by a stranger? He obviously had no idea about what I wanted and told me I was making the wrong decision to continue labouring. 'The same thing is just going to happen again,' he repeated. He seemed to think another emergency Caesarean was inevitable.

I couldn't believe it. I frantically tried to explain to him between ever-intensifying contractions that I didn't want a C-section. He was dismissive, arrogant and adamant that I was doing the wrong thing, especially as he wouldn't be available if I had to have an emergency Caesar later on. I was made to feel as if the hospital's own on-duty anaesthetist, who I would have to use if anything happened—and according to him, it would—was some backyard operator.

I was exasperated. This guy couldn't even wait until a contraction was over to tell me how unfair it would be if he had to be called back late that night and then turn up the next morning to perform an elective Caesar on another woman. It was as if I was not only putting my baby at risk, but also the baby of the woman next on his list.

I went from excitement to desperation in an instant. 'I want to speak with my doctor,' I said as calmly as a labouring woman could. Poor old Fabio didn't know what to do but he kept telling me that it was all going to be okay and we'd sort it out.

The anaesthetist left us stunned, and when I explained everything to my midwife she seemed quite shocked. Later on she said she'd completely misread us and what we wanted to do. She thought we were calm and confident and ready for that early Caesarean when we first arrived at the hospital—not thrilled and relieved that I wouldn't have to have one.

Once I explained everything to her, she was completely on board and turned out to be the voice of reason I needed that night. She got on the phone to my doctor, who said he was happy for me to labour as long as we kept a close eye on the baby. She did an internal and I was three centimetres dilated, the maximum I had ever reached after being induced with Joe.

Then the heart monitor was strapped to my tummy. Everything seemed okay for a while—the contractions were getting increasingly intense and I started throwing up incessantly, which was a lovely feature of my last labour too—until suddenly we watched as the heart rate started to drop into danger zone. *Great*, I thought.

All that dread, fear and uncertainty from Joe's birth immediately returned. We were assured it was quite normal for some fluctuations, but after it settled into a rhythm of drops, the midwife seemed concerned and then suddenly I thought I was risking my baby's life by insisting on a vaginal delivery.

I really felt traumatised and we were so confused. It was as if we had to make this major medical call which we didn't want to make. There was no way we wanted to go through what we went through with Joe—it was so frightening—and I had the anaesthetist's words still ringing in my head. So by about 7.30 p.m. we had pretty much decided to throw it all in for a C-section and called our midwife in to tell her.

She was amazing. She assured us that everything was fine and if it wasn't she'd be on to it straight away. She suggested I disentangle myself from the heart monitor machine for a few minutes, have a shower and then see how I felt.

It was the break I needed. The shower felt great on my bulge and was the perfect distraction, although I was still vomiting all over the bathroom and the contractions were becoming quite unbearable.

By the time I was back on the bed and had the heart monitor strapped on, I decided that if I was going to have to stay hooked up to that machine and be unable to move around to manage the labour, then I might as well have an epidural. And if I needed a C-section later on, then it would already be in.

With my charming original anaesthetist gone for the night, the hospital's on-duty one was called. He was absolutely lovely, albeit a little slow in coming—30 minutes felt like four hours. As he put the needle into my spine, I was expecting instant relief like I had with Joe. But I still felt massive contractions. He topped it up a bit more—they didn't want it too high because if something happened to my Caesarean scar, we all wanted to know about it—and I finally felt numbed. Thank God for epidurals. Heaven.

By now, the baby's heartbeat looked okay and my midwife decided to do another internal. I was eight centimetres dilated and only had two to go. No wonder I still felt those contractions after that first epidural hit.

Rather worryingly, my waters hadn't broken and the baby was still way up high. The baby was also brow-presenting instead of head first, which was not very good, but my midwife said she wasn't going to go near my waters to break them, which turned out to be another great decision of restraint.

Our eyes remained glued to that gloomy monitor but now that the epidural was in, I felt a lot more relaxed. Fabio started to kick back and even turned on the TV to check out what was on. He had no idea. I think he really thought that because the epidural was in, the baby would just slide out and his work was done. Sure thing.

About half an hour later I felt a big rush of water and the baby's head finally moved down. It could have gone either way—brow or crown first. If it were brow, I'd be heading for the operating theatre. Crown, I could stay.

As soon as my midwife did another examination, she started jumping around the room yelling out 'Yes!' as if she'd scored a goal, and ordered Fabio to get the mirror so I could see what was happening. I knew it was crown.

I loved that mirror. To see that beautiful mat of black hair in exactly the right place was just amazing. And somehow I knew it belonged to a little girl.

I was now fully dilated. The epidural was wearing off, I felt like pushing, but my midwife, who said she wasn't going home until this baby was born, told me I had to wait until I felt like doing a big poo. As she went to call my doctor, I looked at that empty baby crib and couldn't believe it was actually going to happen. After last time, it felt strange not to have a full medical entourage ready and waiting.

The baby's heart started to play up again and soon my midwife said the baby really needed to come out. Another midwife appeared and the pushing began. Everybody says giving birth is like pooing a watermelon and it is. As I pushed with my feet pressed into the upper thighs of both my midwives, my baby's little black-haired head would pop out and then go back. Again and again. I focused solely on that mirror.

About half an hour into the push of my life, my obstetrician arrived in gumboots, looking like he was going out for a spot of fishing. He was coaxing me to push but after a while he said, 'I think we might need a little assistance here.' I clearly remember the look my midwife gave him.

I wasn't asked if I wanted an episiotomy, it was just done. I didn't even realise I'd had one until I was about to leave hospital and another midwife checked my stitches and told me that indeed I'd been cut. I didn't really mind, but it would have been nice to be asked.

As I felt a burning sensation in my bottom and continued to push, the baby's chubby cheeks eventually came popping out. 'It's another Joe!' I yelled—those cheeks—and then everyone told me to stop pushing. The umbilical cord was wrapped around the baby's throat, twice, and my doctor smoothly and calmly unravelled it before I started pushing again.

Once her head was out, I couldn't understand it. In wildlife documentaries, baby animals just slithered straight out after the head. Not here. I had to push just as hard to get her body out. Then, when Rosalie appeared just after 10.30 p.m., I understood why. She had her elbow bent and tiny hand up near her shoulder as if she was giving a little wave hello.

I found out later that Fabio had to sit on a stool for support around this time. While I was draining blood from his left hand, he had his head in his right because he thought he'd faint.

Rosalie was whisked away to be checked out and I lay back relieved and exhausted. The first thing I wanted to know was that all her bits were in the right place and doing the things they should, and they were.

The placenta came out and I was happy the mirror was taken away, because my God, it was a mess. I asked my obstetrician how many stitches I'd have to have. 'You don't want to know,' he said. 'But you are going to be pretty sore for a few days.' He was right.

The midwife passed Rosalie to me and I had a good

look at my little girl. She was all squashed up, with red, patchy skin and bloodshot eyes, but she was lovely. I put her to my breast and her little mouth sucked away, and it all came back to me.

I was exhausted but I was in a state of happiness and was as blissed out as I was after Joe's birth. I'd given birth the way I'd wanted and I had my beautiful Rosalie. I also had a story to tell her one day, which would be all her very own. Could have done with those extra days in hospital though.

Postscript

With her two children's birthdays four days apart just weeks before Christmas, Katrina O'Brien dreads the thought of having to decorate two cakes in the same week for the rest of her life.

She always said she'd never have three children if she had to have another Caesarean, but after Rosalie's delivery she'd love to give birth again. It's just the sleepless nights that come afterwards that she's wary of. However, her nausea-prone TV commercial director husband is more than happy with his blue-eyed boy and brown-eyed girl.

Whatever happens, sex is banned in March.

Acknowledgments

My deepest gratitude goes to the women of *Birth Stories*: Alison Baker, Linda Burney, Jenny Ann Cook, Nikki Gemmell, Amanda Keller, Snezna Kerekovic, Penny McCarthy, Sally Machin, Liz Scott, Anne Stanley, Zali Steggall, Kirsty Sword Gusmão and Jane Torley, for their generosity and for being bold enough to share some of the most intimate moments of their lives. Thank you also to the many other women who told me their stories and pointed me in the right direction.

Many, many thanks go to my dear friend, Christine Champion, who appointed herself editorial assistant as soon as I came up with the idea but was much more. Thank you for the unwavering belief, constant encouragement, spot-on insights and the odd chapter title.

Thank you to Hazel Flynn and Sharon Aris, who told me how it could be done. To my lovely sisters Sally Ann and Mary-Louise and Andrea Mariano, Ann Gordon, David Meagher and Tamara Pitelen, who provided very practical support and kept me focused.

Immense thanks to my mother Maureen, father John, and Anna and the Nardos for the non-stop babysitting and dinners and for reminding me that there would be an end.

Thank you to the very clever Jo Paul for taking a risk and making the process so much easier for a novice. Thanks also to Emma Cotter.

To my darling husband, Fabio Nardo, who hardly read a word but did everything else: thank you for still talking to me, and also for our little gems. And finally, a very special thank you to my two best mates Rosalie and Joe, who were my inspiration and are our lives.

About the author

Katrina O'Brien was born in Darlinghurst, Sydney, in 1968. She studied journalism at Mitchell College of Advanced Education in Bathurst and has worked for *Who Weekly*, *Mode*, *Vogue*, Wagga Wagga's *Daily Advertiser*, *Ad News* and *B*, and has edited *Girlfriend*. She is a freelance writer and contributor to *Sunday Life*, and the mother of two young children. *Birth Stories* is her first book.

BIRTH Bir OBr 2005
O'Brien, Katrina
Birth Stories

BIRTH Bir OBr 2005
O'Brien, Katrina
Birth Stories